Transform Your Sex Life:

How to improve your sex life and rediscover the passion with your partner. Sex tips, spanking and domestic discipline. Submissive training and sexy games.

by Paula Ann & Damian Old

Table of Contents

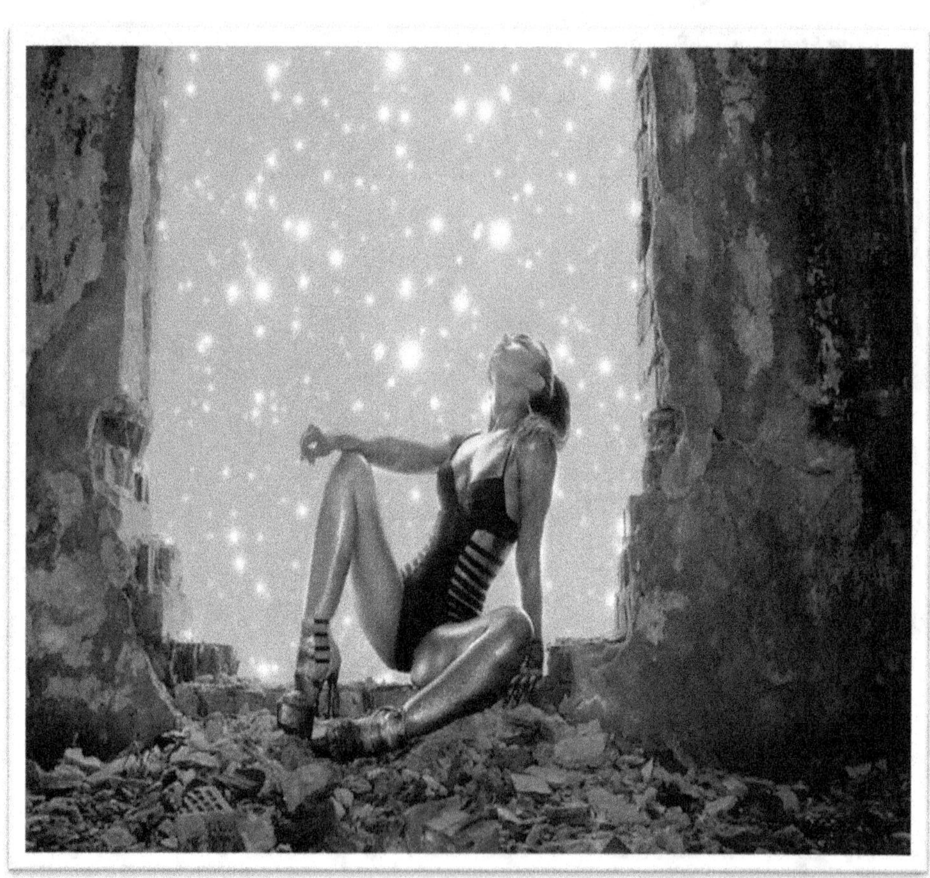

Introduction

Great sex has the power to lift your spirits and make you feel happier. Similarly, bad sex leads to frustration and dissatisfaction. That is why you're here right now. Reading this. You want to enhance the sexual pleasure you and your lover share, and this book is designed to help you do just that. Amazing sex may mean different things to different people, but up skilling your sexual knowledge and venturing beyond your comfort zone is already a step in the right direction.

This book is not just for couples alone, either. Anyone can benefit from the positions covered in this book, even if you're only looking for casual sex until you've found The One. In fact, some of the positions in this book can make casual sex feel carnal and exciting and for the couples who are in relationships, it can bring the fire back into the bedroom as you send each other over the edge with orgasmic experiences that will strengthen your bond as a couple and leave you giddy with pleasure hours after you've had sex.

This book is packed with all you need to know from tips and tricks, beginner, and more advanced sex positions, even an explanation about how to use certain positions to overcome anxiety. We will even explore what introducing sex toys into the bedroom is going to do for your love life and how lube, the unsung hero of the sex world, is going to change your sex life for the better. We will cover the basics and work out way up from there to positions that are going to test your strength and endurance. This book is meant for both men and women, told from the alternating perspectives of both sexes, and you might even read it together as you journey towards better sex like a team.

Intimacy is an important part of every relationship. Getting to know your partner and connecting with them on a deeper level through communication and affection can go a long way to ensuring a relationship grows into a strong and resilient love that can last for decades. While this book primarily focuses on intimacy in new couples, anyone in any type of relationship can apply the principles and suggestions offered here.

Intimacy evolves over time, from intense and frequent to more routine and sometimes infrequent. For this reason, more effort and creativity should be placed, from increasing the spontaneity in your marriage or relationship to creating a surprise for your partner with a new activity or idea.

If you are with a new partner or spouse, it may take time to become comfortable and well acquainted with them. Every situation is different. Some couples progress quickly, while others take their relationship slowly. In every personal relationship, there needs to develop a strong sense of trust and open communication first, as these both serve as a solid foundation for a close, loving bond. When the power of trust and communication is underestimated, challenges and misunderstandings could arise, often leading to unintended difficulties and hurt. Most, if not all, future problems can be averted with a strong desire to communicate and understand the other person's priorities.

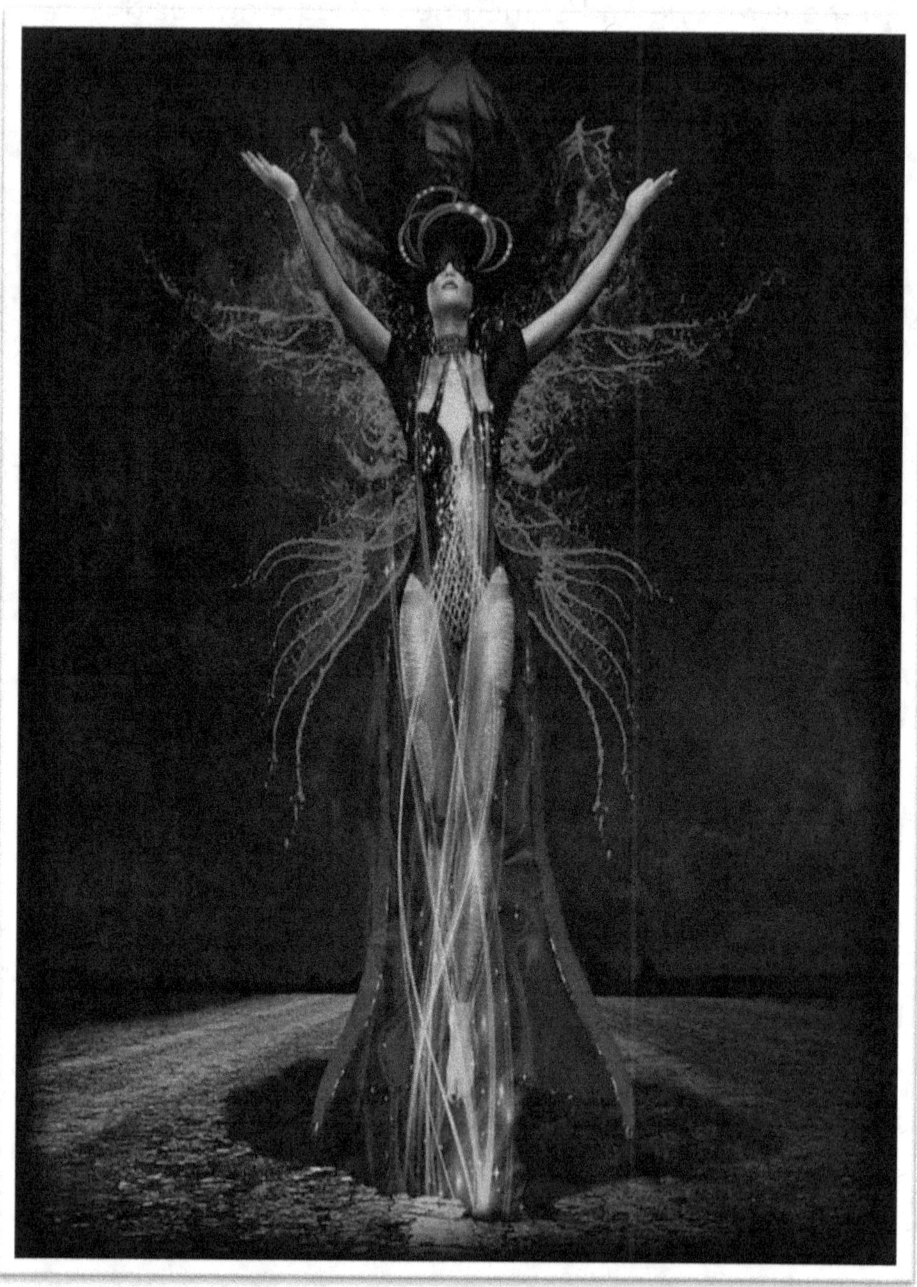

Chapter 1 Transformation

There's nothing like the emotional, happy high that you get from being in a loving, committed relationship. When you're genuinely happy, everything is right with the world, and your lover can do no wrong. The happy glow and the smile on your face can be seen from a mile away. Your family and your friends notice this new positive change about you, now that you have this one special person in your life. You can't believe your good fortune that you've managed to land someone as incredible as your partner.

Is this really happening? Is he/she in love with me? What if they leave me once they realize my flaws?

A healthy and happy relationship that is thriving and going strong can only exist when both partners are comfortable with themselves and with each other. A relationship cannot keep going strong for long if it is filled with doubt and insecurity. The very first question you would probably be asking yourself is, why on earth would I want to subject myself to being hurt that way? That's perfectly understandable. Unless you've already got a boatload of courage buried deep within you, being vulnerable and wearing your heart on your sleeve is going to prove to be a challenge.

Loving Yourself the Most

Trusting someone is something that takes time, but to be able to trust them enough to freely be who you are, you're going to need to open yourself to be vulnerable. What makes this process difficult is that by being completely open and honest in this way, you're leaving the door wide open for the other person to hurt you. For love to blossom, happiness must be a priority. There's no exception to this rule. Couples must love each other despite their flaws, and before you can trust that your partner loves and accepts you for who you are, you need to accept and love yourself. If you find it hard to love and respect yourself, how do you expect anyone else to love you the way you deserve?

Confidence is an attractive quality for both men and women for a reason. When you love yourself, you see your true value. You know what your strengths are and why anyone would be lucky to have you as a partner, so you don't question your lover's motives and wonder what on earth they're doing with you when they could probably be with someone better. Loving yourself means you know what you want and what you're not willing to put up with. You're not going to tolerate anything less than you deserve that threatens to take away your happiness. Put your happiness first, and everything else falls into place, including being in a mutually respectful and loving relationship.

The more you love yourself, the less you will rely on your partner to validate your self-worth. Placing your value in the hands of another is how you become insecure and needy in your relationship. You're so worried your partner is going to find someone else that you're not focused enough on trying to strengthen the relationship. Relinquishing control by seeking validation externally is never going to bring any true happiness and insecurity is a chemistry killer. It won't be long before the initial passion that drew you to each other diminishes when not enough time is being spent nurturing the relationship because your partner is too busy having to reassure you that you're worthy of being loved.

When you love yourself, you know what you want. You know what kind of partner you deserve. You know what you want to get out of your relationship. You know where you want to be several years from now and you're not willing to settle for less than the best. Loving yourself is the best thing you can do for your happiness. Long-lasting happiness needs to come from within. When you're happy with yourself and the life you have, finding someone to share that love and happiness with is a bonus, not a necessity. A man and woman should never rely on each other as the main source of happiness. What happens if that source is gone one day? The only person responsible for your happiness is you and it is the only way to ensure that no matter what happens in your life, you're strong enough to bounce back from it. Even if you lose your relationship.

Understanding Your Sexual Pleasures

Ask anyone what kind of sex they want to have, and they'll tell you they want "great sex." Yet, not everyone can define what "great sex" means to them and there's a very good reason for this. They don't understand their bodies enough. They don't know the way their body reacts and why it reacts the way it does to certain stimuli. They don't know what techniques work best on themselves and their partners. Some might not even be aware of what their erogenous zones are. It's going to be hard to have "great sex" unless you know your body well enough inside at out. So let's get to know your body better:

- Your Erogenous Zones - Essentially, these are the areas of your body with lots of nerve endings that get you aroused or excited when they're touched in the right way. The biggest erogenous zones in the body for most people are the vagina, penis, vulva, labia, clitoris, prostate, perineum, anus, and the scrotum. Out of these, it is generally the clitoris and the penis that are the most sensitive zones. Everyone's body is different, and for some, their erogenous zones might their neck, butt, breasts, thighs, feet, mouth, and nipples. To find out which areas excite you the most, you need to experiment until you hit the sweet spot (or your partner does).

- The Sex Cycle Response - This describes the way that your body reacts when it is sexually stimulated. This cycle could either happen alone or with your partner. The sex cycle happens in several stages. The first stage is desire, where thinking sexual thoughts begin to arouse and excite you, getting your body primed and ready for sex. The second stage of the cycle is the plateau stage, and you're fully aroused by this point, ready to either have sex or masturbate. The third and final stage of the cycle is the orgasm phase when all that sexual tension that has been building up is finally released and your body convulses with pleasure.

- Explore Your Body - It's time to get intimate with yourself if you haven't done that already. Before you can understand what turns you on, you need to give yourself an anatomy lesson. Learn to please your body through self-stimulation and exploration. It's okay to be nervous about this in the beginning, touching yourself intimately in that way may feel strange and unfamiliar at first. Take your time exploring yourself thoroughly, so you know what turns you on and what causes discomfort. Our understanding of our bodies affects your mindset and the more comfortable you are with your body, the easier it will be to succumb to the pleasure when you're with your lover.

- Understanding Orgasms - Sexual stimulation doesn't need to happen to experience an orgasm. Most couples would be surprised to know this. There are a few ways to define what an orgasm means. Medical professionals think of it as the physiological change that the body undergoes. Psychologists see it as your body experiencing cognitive and emotional changes. At the moment, there's no overarching description that succinctly depicts what an orgasm means, but what we do know is that it feels extremely good when it happens. Orgasms have a few categories too. Multiple orgasms, G-spot orgasms, fantasy orgasms, relaxation orgasms, tension orgasms, and a combination of the different experiences coming together. Which one you experience depends on the context in which it is happening.

Sexuality is a constant state of exploration.

Depending on how comfortable you are and how long you've been in a relationship, you'll be curious, pushing your boundaries and exploring just how far you can go. We evolve and grow with time, and so does our sexuality. It's not a permanent state of being. It's a work in progress, one that you must give yourself time to adjust to. Your body is a source of pleasure and it is time you got to know that.

The Way to Better Female Orgasms

Pleasure is different for everyone and you shouldn't believe everything that you watch in porn. Getting an orgasm is a unique experience for each woman and it is still very much an area of mystery for both sexes. Believe it or not, women don't need to climax to be sexually happy and satisfied by their lovers. Too much pressure is placed on women achieving orgasm the way a man does, which is practically at every sexual encounter. Men feel pressured when their partner doesn't orgasm, and it makes him question his capabilities, while women feel pressured enough to fake an orgasm because they don't want to disappoint their partners. This might have something to do with the innate fear we all have about being "rejected" if we fail to live up to the sexual expectations placed upon us. Needless to say, this is going to be an orgasm killer for many women.

Not helping matters is the taboo that has been surrounding the subject of women and self-exploration for a long time. The notion that "good girls" don't touch themselves in that way has made many of us feel uncomfortable and even ashamed of our natural desires. Female sexual pleasure is one of the least talked about subjects, but it is a subject you need to start embracing. Sexual satisfaction can only be achieved (alone or with your partner) when you know what works for you.

- Take as much time as you need getting to know your body. Don't be afraid to use your fingers and a couple of toys during your exploration process.

- Explore stimulating and putting pressure on your clitoris and see how you feel.

- Touch your body all over when you're in the shower and explore every inch and hidden crevice in detail. It's an exercise in getting to know your various body parts.

- Wear a blindfold when you masturbate alone and let your other senses come alive to replace the one that has been temporarily taken aware. This heightened sensitivity makes you aware of what stimulation gets you off the most.

- Follow good old-fashioned advice and grab a mirror and look at yourself down there.

- Explore stimulating your clitoris, vagina, vulva and the surrounding area with your fingers or with sex toys if you prefer. Try different strokes, positions, and varying degrees of pressure to see what brings you closer to the big O.

Postponing Your Ejaculation

Nature made is such that women are fortunate enough to experience prolonged orgasms that come in waves. A man's orgasm, on the other hand, is brief but explosive, lasting anywhere from 5-7 seconds at a time. Men would love if this feeling could last longer than a couple of seconds no doubt, but so far, there's no tried and true method to keep the orgasm going for longer. One study reveals that between the age of 18 and 60, at least 30% of men within this age group will prematurely ejaculate at some point. It may not always happen, but when it does, it is characterized as ejaculation happening within a minute of penetration most of the time.

The good news is, there are ways you can delay it. You may not be able to prolong the sensation, but you can prolong the pleasure and delay the orgasm enough so you last longer.

To delay what inevitably is going to happen, a man needs to get as close to the threshold as possible, and then halt. Stop the stimulation, breathe, and relax all the muscles around the lower back and perineum. Wait until the sensation has passed before you begin the stimulation again. It sounds easy enough in theory, but it takes considerable effort, mental and emotional discipline, and a lot of willpower for him to pull himself back from the brink of sexual bliss. The trick to making this technique work is to reach the highest state of excitement right before he is about to ejaculate and then forcibly pull back. By withholding himself from the pleasure, he is opening the door for even greater levels of excitement the next time he is stimulated. Keep the cycling going by reaching high and then pulling back as many times as possible until he can finally take no more. The best way to practice this technique is when you're masturbating alone. Do what you would normally do to self-stimulate, come close, and then pull back. See how many times you can repeat the process until you finally release all that pent up energy and ejaculate with gusto.

Other techniques you could try include:

- Squeeze It - To bring your happy ending to a halt, try squeezing the shaft of your penis right before you're about to ejaculate. Give it a good squeeze between your thumb and forefinger, but to the point where it's causing you pain. The act of squeezing it is going to minimize your erection slightly so you can

spend more time going at it with your
partner.

- The Diversion - When you're about to reach
  your peak, let your mind wander and distract
  it from the sensation that you feel in your
  nether regions. Distraction and diversion shift
  your mind and your body away from the
  focus of peaking too early.

- Breathe Deeply - To successfully mitigate
  your ejaculation, breathe from your
  diaphragm when you're making love to your
  partner. This technique is referred to as
  "diaphragm breathing" or "belly breathing."
  When you're about to come, your breathes
  tend to be shorter, sharp, and shallow which
  will cause your heart rate to spike. By
  controlling your breathing with deep,
  measured, in and out breaths, you're actively
  regulating the sensations you feel through
  mindful awareness, allowing you to focus on
  controlling your ejaculation.

- Spray It to Delay It - If all else fails, there's
  always the option of using topical sprays to
  help you delay the process. These sprays are

applied at least 10-minutes prior to sex and directly on the penis. Spritz it a couple of times, and you'll be ready to go strong for the next 30 minutes or so. Maybe even 60 minutes for some men.

The Man's Secret to Multiple Orgasms

It's not a myth. Women are not the only ones capable of multiple orgasms. The man's secret to doing the same lies in a gland that is no bigger than the size of a walnut. Your prostate. When stimulated enough, a man is more than capable of achieving a full-blown orgasm, even if he is not fully erect to do it. The only thing is a lot of straight men might find this uncomfortable since to get to the prostate, they or their partners will have to access it through the anus or alternatively, under the perineum area. But once they get past that initial apprehension though, everything changes,

A lot of straight men struggle with the idea of letting their partners stimulate their anus. They're even more uncomfortable with having to do it themselves. This hang-up has more to do with the mindset than anything else. Enjoying the pleasure of anal stimulation has nothing to do with what your sexual preference may be. It takes a man who is open-minded enough to get past this way of thinking, and if it means you now have access to the secret of multiple orgasms, why not?

If you are attempting this by yourself or with your partner, use a lot of water-based lube to avoid hurting the sensitive tissue around the area. You can either do this by yourself or with your partner. When you're ready, gently slide your lubed-up finger into your anus. Allow your body time to get comfortable with the sensation and then begin to angle your finger towards the direction of your penis. Once you feel slight pressure, that's when you know you've found the right spot. It's going to feel a little like you have to pee before the sensation begins to shift from intense pleasure to oh-my-god orgasmic bliss.

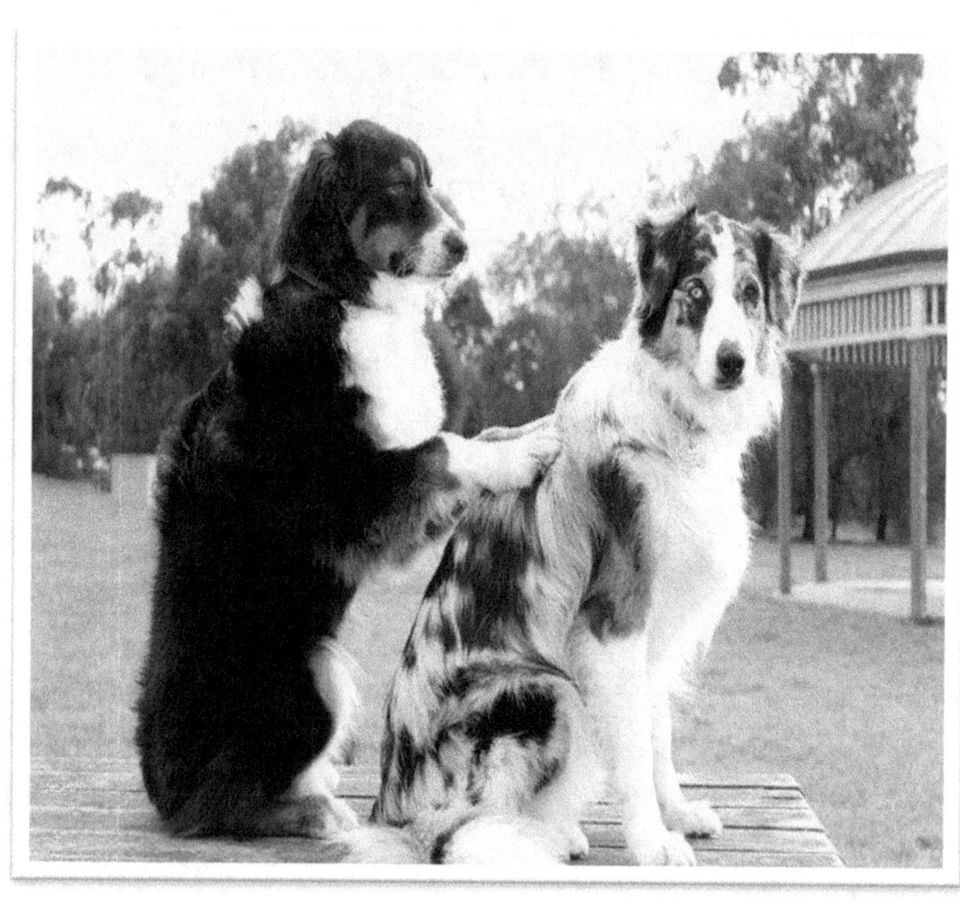

Chapter 2 Physical And Mental Benefits Of Sex

Here we are going to talk about sexual chemistry and sexual intuition. Sexual chemistry is a conglomeration of signs and signals that help us understand if we are sexually compatible with another person or not. It is something our bodies tell us, not our brains, and it cannot be denied. Sexual intuition and sexual chemistry go hand in hand.

We will start by discussing sexual chemistry. Sexual chemistry can be difficult to define, but we will do our best. It is the way our body understands attraction and love without our minds being involved. When you are around someone, and you feel as if a shock runs through your body, it is our body's way of showing us there is chemistry. This occurs because of sexual intuition.

Intuition, in itself, is when we can understand something right away without our conscious playing any sort of role in it. These are our feelings of instinct. Intuition helps us know when we are in danger or in a place of safety. It helps clue us into the intention of the world around us.

The attraction we feel toward someone before we know anything about them is another good way to describe sexual chemistry. It's that magnetism that can simply not be ignored. Sometimes it can be quite overwhelming, while other times, it feels like a simple tug.

Many times, when sexual chemistry is high, it will feel as if you have no control over yourself. Your desire for that individual will overrule your head. It sweeps over people quickly and cannot be denied. It can happen from a look, a touch, or even their voice. You never know what the thing will be that shows you have great sexual chemistry with another person.

When people say they feel "fireworks" when they kiss someone for the first time, it is a sign of good sexual chemistry. The desire you experience with high levels of sexual chemistry will be unlike what you have experienced before. It will feel more like a need rather than a want.

It is hard for some people to accept that our bodies could know something so important before our brains have time to analyze it; however, it is true. One of the first things to help us understand that a person is fit to be in a relationship with is sexual chemistry and intuition. Our bodies are drawn to those that we are compatible with. Likewise, if someone is a terrible fit for us, we are often times put off or repelled by their mere presence. Paying attention to what your body is telling you can help you make sound decisions when looking for a lover.

You do need to be mindful of the type of chemistry you are experiencing. It could be simple lust as you are attracted to a certain look or body type. You need to pay attention to the cues that you are receiving from the inside. Are you actually interested in getting to know the person you are looking at, or are you simply visualizing what it would be like to take them to bed?

We all have a type, and figuring out what it is that makes up your type is important. Some of it will come from the culture you were raised in, your family, and even your peers. Other pieces of it are not consciously decided but something that is on a deeper level. When we are young, we go through stages where arousal starts. This arousal can leave an imprint on us that will stay with us throughout our entire lives. When we are young, we don't often realize that we are aroused, but as we get older, certain features in people that struck our fancy when young will become arousing and provide us with sexual stimulation. These are frequently physical features like eye color, hair type, and physical build.

These imprints can come from a variety of different things. Oftentimes it happens when we see something sexual in nature for the first time, such as pornography. The desire we feel gets burned into us and can sometimes help to explain personal fantasies and even some fetishes.

The intense sexual chemistry that you feel for another person can absolutely just be lust related to the sexual imprints we gather when we are younger. This is oftentimes recognized and typically ends up in limited time spent together. These encounters can help fulfill a want or desire, but your body lets your brain know that it is nothing more than a hookup.

There are many times that people ignore what their bodies are telling their minds and allow lust to become a relationship. Sometimes it works out and other times, not so much. Lust is a good thing to have, but it doesn't usually lead to a fulfilling relationship. It takes more than lusting after someone to be able to sustain and find a healthy relationship.

When you start to crush on someone, there are definitely signs to show you if there is a good level of sexual chemistry or not. Paying attention to the signs can help you make better choices when you are choosing a partner. The signs can show you if there is a future between the two of you or if it will end up being a bust.

When you start to get to know a person if you feel like everything is forced, it is likely that you don't have very good sexual chemistry. It should not feel forced when you have good sexual chemistry things will come naturally. So, if you are not really feeling the other person's vibe, you should certainly pay attention to it and probably start looking at different options.

It is important to note that sometimes, first meetings can be awkward. So, judging your level of chemistry after the first date may not be the best course of action. It is normal for a first date to be a bit rocky, give your intended a chance even if you find that things are a bit difficult on the first go. After the second or third date, if it still feels forced and awkward, it is probably time to move on and find a new avenue for a relationship.

As you are feeling things out, you will gain a better understanding of if it is going to work or not. Oftentimes, things will start to go a bit smoother as you start to get to actually know someone. You can actually work on your chemistry if it lacks in the beginning if you think the person you are spending time with is worth it.

Reading the signs when there is initial sexual chemistry is actually pretty easy if you know what you are looking for. One good sign is when the person you are with leans toward you when you are interacting. Conversely, if they are angling themselves away from you, it is a good sign that your chemistry is not that good.

You should also pay attention to how you feel when you make eye contact with the person you are thinking of entering into a relationship with. Eye contact can be hard to maintain, but the feeling it gives you when there is good sexual chemistry will not fill you with anxiety or the inane need to instantly look away. The ability to hold eye contact is a good sign that you are compatible with the person you are seeing.

Nerves play a major role in whether or not you will be able to maintain contact for more than a second or two. So, don't judge someone too harshly if they can't hold eye contact for very long on a first date. It is completely normal; however, if it continues to be difficult after a few dates, it is a pretty clear sign that things are not going so well, and the person you are seeing is likely not the one for you.

The interaction that takes place between you and your intended is one of the biggest signs of how the chemistry is between the two of you. They want to make physical contact with someone, and the way you act around each other will be good tells as to how things are going. Your awareness of each other will be more tuned in than it is with other people. Things will not feel forced.

The movements of a couple that has excellent sexual chemistry will be fluid. It will be like they have been around each other for a long period of time, even if they have only had a few encounters. The way they interact and move will be easy; it will be as if they don't need to try because they have been doing it all along regardless of the time frame of knowing each other.

Communication is a key element in a successful relationship. When you are able to talk to someone easily from the word go, it is a very good sign. Feeling as if you can tell someone the truth about who you are, where you come from, and what your wants, needs, and desires are is rare, and it should be cherished. If someone can open up to you the same way, it is a pretty clear sign that you should continue on with them and see where things go.

Everyone has heard the phrase, "Go with your gut!" and there is certainly truth behind it. Our gut instinct is there for a reason, and it can give you great insight into whether or not you are compatible and likely have good sexual chemistry with another person. When you are simply near someone, do you find yourself wanting to move closer and touch them? Maybe you feel as if you can't wait to get out of there. Either way, your gut is trying to tell you something, and you should listen.

When you start to look at all of these aspects, it really does help us to understand when we have good sexual chemistry with someone. More often than not, you want it to happen naturally. As with all things in life, you should give every situation a shot as anxiety, stress, and nerves can all play a role in initial meetings.

Once in a while, you will meet someone, and it will start off as a hit, but over the course of time, things will dwindle. You may notice that the sexual chemistry that you used to possess has gone to the wayside. No need to worry, there are things you can do to help boost your sexual chemistry. You can:

- Put some time and distance between the two of you. Remember that distance makes the heart grow fonder.
- Add romance to the relationship by planning special dates, leaving love notes, or bringing a surprise gift home.
- Experiment with new things in the bedroom.
- Take time to remember what it is about your partner that you truly love and appreciate.

- Express to your partner what they mean to you and why.

These are only a couple of the things you can do to spice up a relationship and get your sexual chemistry back to where it used to be. Relationships are work, so keeping this kind of thing going simply needs you to pay attention to it. If things aren't going quite right or you feel like something is off, you should start by talking with your partner about it. Then you can brainstorm together and figure out what to do together to fix any issues that may arise.

There are many things in life that our intuition tells us, it is a matter of paying attention to the intuitions. There are some that you should absolutely not ignore as they help you understand sex and love better than you might think. Paying attention to the subtleties of life can really help us along our path in trying to find true love and a relationship that will last.

We have discussed several feelings or signs that you should not ignore, but there are a few more that are important. Have you ever had the feeling of déjà vu? You know those moments in life that you feel as if you have experienced them before. That you could say or predict what is about to happen next. Realistically it is impossible to know what someone is about to say or what is going to happen once you turn the corner. Still, it happens to us all.

When instances of déjà vu occur, we absolutely need to pay attention to them. Rather than chalking it up to a strange occurrence, take some time and review it. Talk it out with a friend or even take the time to put it in a journal. With reflection, déjà vu can help us see more clearly and, in turn, make better decisions.

Within your romantic relationship, déjà vu can help you confirm if you are on the right track or if you need to be looking for a new mate. When we experience this occurrence, it can show us the context of our relationships. It can provide us with the knowledge of what fuels the relationship and how significant it is in the grand scheme of our own individual paths. As you can see, déjà vu is not a thing to be ignored.

One last intuition that is really important to pay attention to and can help us understand if someone is compatible with us in a sexual and relationship nature is synchronicity. Synchronicity is when you have a sense that something or someone has perfect timing. When you have been singing a song to yourself and all of a sudden, it pops on the radio, or you run into someone you once hand a crush on at the coffee shop.

Synchronicity can be seen easily if you are looking for it. When you are at the moment of being in the right place at the right time, utilize it. Look for the significance in the experience. Not only can it clue you into things that are right, but it can also show you when things are about to go wrong. What was the name of that song stuck in your head that played on the radio? Was it about love or the loss of it? By asking yourself questions like this, you can frequently come to a better understanding of where things are going.

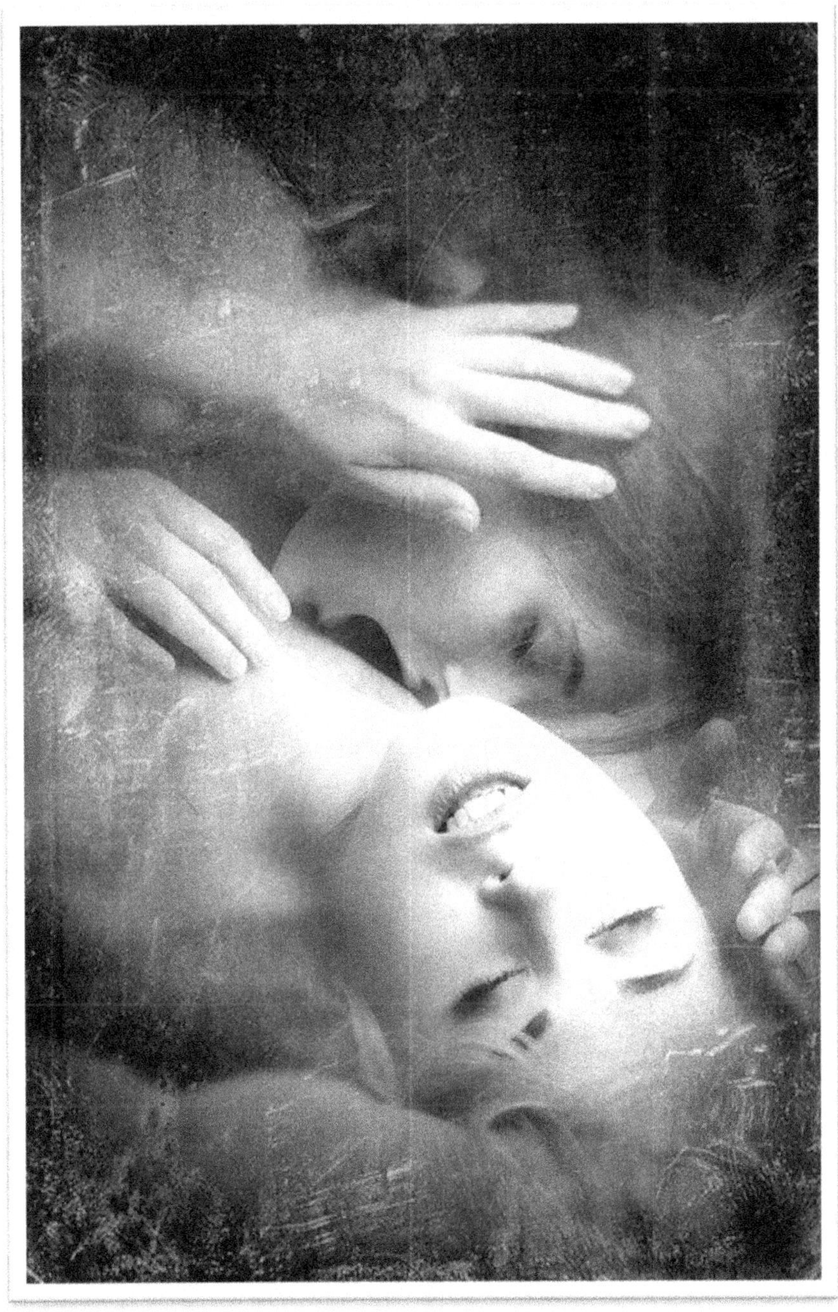

Chapter 3 Understanding TheComplexity Between Pleasure And Orgasm

Powerful Sex Positions for Male Orgasm

If you want to help your man achieve orgasm and pleasure, you must understand his level of thrill in orgasm. Most women do not know that male orgasm differs in intensity depending on various factors. Therefore, women should not try out similar ways to impress different men. Similarly, they should understand the positions that their men like and those that they do not. There are various things to do to encourage a bone-rattling orgasm from your man. Notably, the endeavor to impress your man may be involving surprises and contradictions hence the expected complications. The fact that men are sensitive to technique and skill makes them easily powered by setting, timing, and mood. Therefore, you need to incorporate one or all of the following sex positions to help your man get a longer and stronger orgasm.

Missionary- In this position, the man is usually on top, and the woman lies on her back on a flat platform. There are various variations of this position, and all are fit to cause a powerful orgasm for your man. The position enhances eye contact making it easy for the man to read facial expressions and make sexy gestures on his face. The reaction of the woman gives the man a sexy impression making it easy to reach orgasm. The position also leaves the man to be in control of the depth, pace, and angle of penetration, making him feel dominant over the woman. It also allows the man to adjust, especially if he decides to include variations of the missionary position. Some of these variations will enable the woman to close her legs, closing up the groin and tightening the vagina. The intense sensitivity from the narrow vagina gives the man a mind-blowing orgasm. In this position, the man may use his hands to caress the woman making him explore additional benefits from the activity. As a result, the man feels satisfied and may ejaculate due to the overwhelming pleasure.

Cowgirl- Also known as the woman on top, this position has the woman on top and the man lying on his back on a flat platform. It is known to allow the woman to control most aspects that are involved, such as depth and speed of penetration. Nevertheless, the position is known to turn men on due to the eye contact maintained, especially if the partners are facing each other. Similarly, variations of this position enable the woman to make different angles meant to stimulate the man. By closing her legs, the woman makes the area tight, creating more friction that enhances orgasm and possible ejaculation. It also allows the woman to lay her hands on the man's chest or stomach and combine sexual stimulation with caressing. The man's hands are also free to reach the woman's clit or nipples to make the activity realistic. The sense of touch, in this case, enhances the man's orgasm making it most preferable sex position. If the woman decides to turn and face the same direction as the man eye, contact is reduced, making the man lose his self-consciousness and achieve pleasure consciousness. He is taken into his fantasies, creating a powerful orgasm inevitable. The girl on top position is known to work best for men with problems controlling their orgasm. It gives men time to relax and under little pressure making it possible to maintain and prolong their orgasm.

Doggy- The doggy style involves men penetrating from behind. Similar to other positions, this one too has variations that allow a change in angles and posture. Men admire the position as it gives them the notion of being dominant than the female. When a woman bends over in the doggy style, the man may choose to sit, stand, or kneel behind her. The posture gives men more comfort and ease of access. They can leverage the power they apply to penetrate, making them attain speedy orgasm due to the effort they use. The balance that men have in this position makes it easy for them to dominate the activity and enjoy as the woman finds support elsewhere. If the man decides to stand, kneel, or sit, he still can caress the woman as his hands remain relaxed, making it possible to reach the hair, nipples, or the clitoris. The position exposes the woman's genitals, making it visible for the man to assess the activity and find pleasure in it. By watching the action take place, the man could indulge in a powerful orgasm. The inability of the man to make eye contact or read facial expressions makes him into fantasies that are mostly influenced by the sense of touch and imagination. Doggy style has numerous variations where the man is free to make adjustments on his depth and speed of penetration, leaving him with all the pleasure he yearns. Each partner supports themselves, leaving the man comfortable. The weight is supported on his feet, allowing him to direct all his efforts to the activity.

Spooning-The couples lie on top of each other or on sideways to allow the man to penetrate the woman from behind as the bodies stretch out on a flat platform. The woman may lift one of her legs to allow easy penetration. The position provides a powerful male orgasm, primarily due to the full body contact associated with it. Both partners enjoy the cuddling that comes along with a sweet penetration. The hands are left free, making the man access the clitoris or her nipples. It appears simple and requires little effort since all partners have their bodies supported. Besides, the couples remain relaxed as they make variations of the position. It is an ideal position for tired men who may be exhausted for a more complicated position, especially after work. Similarly, it is a preferable morning activity where couples start off the day with fewer efforts and still enjoy. Notably, the friction caused by the buttocks as the man finds his way to the vagina provides a double stimulation for men.

X-rated- As the name suggests, this position involves making an x shape as you engage in sexual intercourse. The man holds the woman's legs full as he moves between them to penetrate. Most of the time, the woman' feet remain wide opened or tangled around the man's waist. It also makes it simple for the man to access the vagina and stimulate the clit. The upper part of the woman's body lies on a flat platform reducing the weight that the man should support. This position enhances penetration for it brings the man close to the genitals putting the feet wide open hence removing possible obstructions. With deep penetration, the man is sure to be meeting his partner's sexual desires making him more stimulated to orgasm and possibly ejaculation. The proximity of the groins makes it simple for the man to make quick thrusts as he hits the partner's genitals. Easy access stimulates men to the genital area of their partner and is impressed mostly by the feeling of touch. Similarly, they can observe the woman's reaction to deep penetration and clit stimulation. This observation turns them on and acts as a catalyst for their orgasm.

It also allows the men to adjust the depth of penetration. The x rated position helps the man hold the woman in a fixed position and decreasing her movements to make a firm and consistent thrust. Besides, a man can control the angle, pace, and depth of his penetration as he is in full control of the activity. The body contact primarily through the woman's thighs makes him feel aroused and given all of it.

Powerful Sex Positions for Female Orgasm

If your woman has difficulties achieving an orgasm, there are certain factors that you need to consider to turn the tide. As with men, women also have different preferences when it comes to what works best for them. For that reason, you should learn to observe the reaction of your partner as you engage in different sex positions. Most women achieve orgasm spending on how their partner stimulates them physically and psychologically. You should start easy as you advance by providing feedback to each other about the comfort, ease, and sensitivity of every stimulation. The following positions are among the best in giving your woman a powerful orgasm

*Missionary:*It is the most comfortable position that you could try out with your partner as she lies on a flat platform. It provides comfort to the woman who is on the receiving end, leaving the man to do most of the work. The woman feels soothed and adored as she gets stimulated by the man's moves.Similarly, the man would utilize his freedom in making hand gestures or caressing the woman as he maintains the thrusts. By just putting his hands on the woman, the man ensures that the partners enjoy the feeling. He could use the hands to stimulate the clitoris, which is positioned right in front of him to give the woman total stimulation of the genitals. This form of stimulus could be combined with that of the nipples to turn the woman wild. The missionary position enhances direct eye contact of the partners. The man can read the woman's facial expression as they create a visual bond and make the exercise more realistic. The woman coordinates the visual effects with the thrusts putting her into a world of pleasure in intimacy. There are variations of this position that allow the man to lie on the woman entirely. This way, the woman experiences full body contact of the man giving her a sense of love and belonging. The posture also enhances the stimulation of the clitoris as the man moves up and down. Other variations of the missionary position allow the woman to cross her legs and make her vagina narrower. The effect makes the man's thrust more solid, increasing the level of stimulation that the woman receives. The friction of the penis and the vaginal walls causes the effect. It would be advisable to encourage a female partner to try out different variations of the missionary position as it the simplest and allows for varied level of stimulation.

*Spooning:*In this position, the man penetrates from behind as both stretches on a flat platform. It is a superior position for a dominant female orgasm as it allows the man to cuddle her with the free hands. The partners should be close together to avoid the penis from slipping out hence the provision of tight contact and access to other body parts. This position ensures that the couples have full body contact and arouses women the feeling of a male body on top of them. They develop a sense of love as they can feel every part of their body and tell the pace from the man's breath and moves. The couples may decide to lie on a bed to avoid one of them holding the total weight. The posture makes this position easy and relaxing to the woman as she lies by her side and lets the man penetrate. The stimulation is influenced by the fact that the man requires no extra effort to satisfy her sexually. The fact that couples face the same direction in this position makes it hard for them to maintain eye contact. Therefore, they make fantasies of their own as they feel the thrusts. In this case, you achieve ultimate orgasm from the enhancement of the sense of touch.

*Woman on Top:*This position allows the woman to take full control of the activity. She ensures that she receives stimulation at the right time and manner. This provision makes it easy for the woman to achieve orgasm as she gets what she wants. The variations of this position allow lying on her man leading to the proximity of the clitoris and the pelvis. As a result, she experiences full body contact of her partner, thus stimulating her sexually and quickening orgasm. It may also enhance a strong erection from the man who eventually would lead to more vaginal stimulation. The position also improved direct eye contact between the woman and her partner. It makes them read each other's facial expressions or make gestures that would enhance orgasm. With the sense of sight being active, the woman feels aroused by reality. The hands of both partners could also freely move around each other's body. This way, the man could reach the woman's nipples, neck, or the clitoris to combine his penetration with caressing. The woman could do the same as she aims to self-stimulate and enhances the performance of the man. By stimulating her partner, the woman enjoys the intimacy and is most likely to reach orgasm. The woman on top position is versatile and allows partners to explore different ways in which they could customize it to reach orgasm. Therefore, you should ensure that you explore various forms of this position to achieve the desired results. You should also give your woman an orgasm that she will always long to have. For instance, you could raise one of your thighs as she performs a reversed position to stimulate her clit. She holds on the knee as she moves back and forth with the penis deep inside her. These variants also allow for self-stimulation in women. They may feel themselves better than their partners and find it better to stimulate their body as they keep the penis penetrated. Self-stimulation mostly happens with the use of sex toys where women achieve orgasm by having sex as they encourage other parts. The woman on top positions also plays a significant role in maintaining and prolonging orgasm for men.Consequently, women have ample time to make fun and enjoy the erect penis. They find it pressurizing to have sex with erectile might and can hold it for a long time. These reasons should encourage you to explore your woman's orgasm through variations of this position.

Doggy: The doggy style involves penetration from behind and has women bending over on a platform. It is a position you could use to get a powerful orgasm from your female partner for the penis lands on the G spot, which is key to orgasm. By frequently rubbing the spot, you sexually stimulate your woman, making her go wild and achieve an orgasm. If the woman leans on a support platform, then she feels relaxed and has less work other than feeling the stimulation form the thrusts. The relaxed mode enables the woman to indulge in the activity both physically and psychologically, making it possible to achieve an orgasm. The position leaves the man's hands available for continued caressing or stimulating either the nipples or the clitoris. This combination enhances sexual sensitivity making the woman experience high degree orgasm and possible ejaculation. The doggy style leaves both the anus and the vagina stimulated. It makes it possible for a man to make deep penetration to reach the rarely accessed points of the woman's vagina. Consequently, the woman gets aroused by the deep penetration giving her a sexy stimulation and eventual orgasm. The man could also practice different angles to ensure that he gets the best out of it as the woman indulges in pleasure fantasies. The animalistic nature of this position adds to its sexiness as most women like it like that.

How to Use Your Hands

How you make your sex drive determines whether your partner enjoys sex. Partners find it hard to keep up with the poor performance of their partners in bed. Various factors, such as stress, make partners hard to turn on. As a result, couples lose their meaning and value in intercourse, making it happen rarely enjoyable. Therefore, you should learn how to spice things up and create an intimate and relaxing environment. With essential tools, there are ways you could transition your partner from being stressed to blissed. It is possible to use your readily available hands to achieve great sexual satisfaction for you and your partner. However, you should understand how to do it to avoid backlash and counter-productivity. The following are ways you could apply your hands and create wild sensation to your partner.

1. *Stimulate Your Partner-* The soft touches that you make to your partner mean a lot to them for it shows connectivity as well as boosting their sexual consciousness. You should ensure that your partner feels you as you caress them and make sensitive touches that arouse them sexually. Your hands are a powerful tool that could turn your partner on if done appropriately and suggestively. The stimulation could be done before, during, and after sexual intercourse as long as it happens with moderation. If your partner has the body covered most of the time, they will enjoy to when hands reach the places that are usually covered.

2. *Guidance-* Most of the sex positions involve partners lying on the bed or being in a

position that leaves only the hands free. They provide an ample opportunity for you to communicate with your partner. Your hands are the best tools to guide your partner in areas that are most stimulating and how to touch them. Men use their hands to hold the woman's head as they receive oral to guide them on the depth and pace. Similarly, you may use your hand to keep your partner's head as you kiss. This way, you are sure to get the best out of it.

3. *Self-stimulation-* It is yet another way to make yourself appreciative and making fun of the moment. Sexual stimulation is not only achieved by the touch of your partners but also your contact. You could use your hands to stimulate your body by working on the nipples or the clitoris. The self-stimulation is regarded as accurate for you know the parts that cause much stimulation as well as how you should caress them. Similarly, you are aware of the limitation to that stimulation as opposed to external stimulation which cannot tell when you have

enough of it. Self-Stimulation makes it possible to reach spots that your partner cannot primarily in a complicated position.

4. *Achieve orgasm-* It has become common among couples to use their hands to achieve inevitable orgasm. Most couples find the hands so sensitive to their genitals that they must be used to help the orgasm. Your soft hand could turn and reach hidden spots in your partner's genital are if only they guide you on the stimulation they need. You could use your fingers to penetrate the vagina and reach the G spot, which could turn the woman wild and wanting. The same mechanism could be applied in case of anal sex to stimulate the nerve endings.

5. *Control-* Much of these controls occurs during sexual intercourse. It is common in the cowgirl, missionary, and the doggy sex positions. As a dominant partner in these positions, you could use your hands to control the movement of your partner as well as bringing them closer to the action. Besides, your hands are vital in controlling

the depth and pace of the penetration for a best intimate session. In cowgirl, you make her move horizontally helps control your point of ejaculation while enhancing the contact of your pelvis with that of the clitoris. You could also change the partner's posture using your hands for a more pleasuring sexual act. Women like to wrap their sides around the man's waist to enhance the pace and help them make a deep penetration.

6. *Utilizing Sex Toys*- You would not want to live all your sex life without having to try sex toys. Most probably, you have already tried a number of them and realized the pleasure associated with them. There are different types of sex toys, and most have various forms of application even though they may appear identical. Besides, you should perfect on the usage of each sex toy before trying it on your partner to avoid mess and embarrassment. Your hands are then the essential tools when it comes to how effective a sex toy is. You should have a firm

grip on the object to ensure that it meets its desired objectives. During sexual intercourse, you should involve sex toys, especially for foreplay and maintenance of sexual stimulation. Your hands should act as the support and director of the toy as it is busy stimulates the sensitive parts of your partner.

7. *Demonstration*- At times, partners do not get what they want due to lack of providing feedback. You should be free to each other on what works best for you and what does not. If your partner does not get what you are asking for, you could use your own hands to show them what they should do to impress you sexually. It includes touching your sensitive parts that your partner may be missing or showing them the pace with which to land on them. You could perform a session they watch to understand what they need to correct and what to expect in every move they make. For instance, you could masturbate to show your partner how you

want them to or how easy it is for you to reach orgasm.

8. *Support*-Most sex positions require couples to be in postures that require them to use hands for support. These are positions that would be suitable for physically fit couples. For instance, the missionary position requires the man to use his hands for help as he penetrates the partner. Numerous variants of sex positions leave only the hands suspended with the other part of the body fixed in a non-supportive place. Partners may also use their hands as pillows to raise their heads or buttock for clear vision or penetration. The support that your hands provide makes you comfortable while enhancing the strength, depth, and pace of the penetration. In the 69 positions, the hand's aid in ensuring that the genitals are easily accessible and serviceable. The support provided in missionary position ensures that the man focuses on stimulation penetration.

You should not let your sex life to lose value and test due to inefficiency caused by how you go down on your partner. Take a step of reshaping your sex life by incorporating additional sexual moves and techniques. These ideas will help shape your relationship as you explore some of the insights provided. They will also help you learn more about your partner and understand what works best for them.

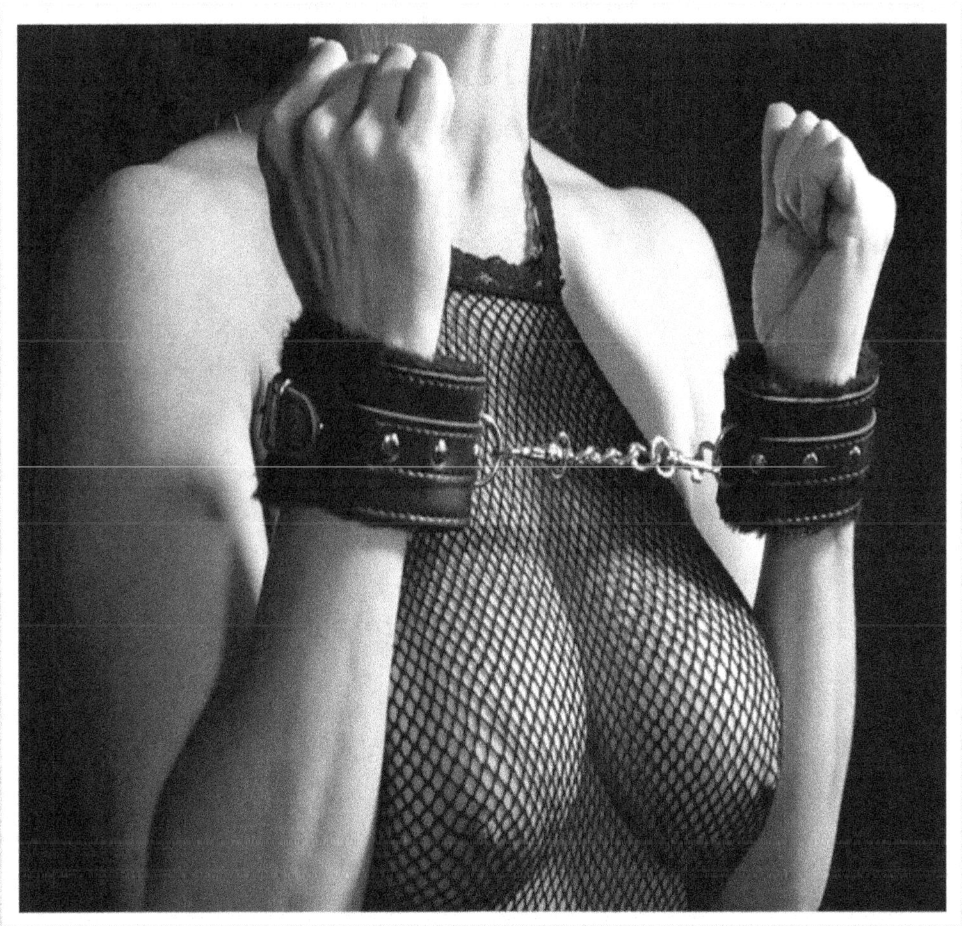

Chapter 4 Picking the Perfect Sex Toys and Fantasies

Now that we have established the details of how sex toys can help you rejuvenate your sex life, we are going to talk about the key ways by which you can pick the right ones. As there is so much variety when it comes to sex toys, it can often be difficult to pick the right one. Not all of them are useful and at the same time, the onus should always be on picking the ones which are sure to help you enjoy the good times in bed.

So, are you set for the ultimate guide who will help you pick the perfect sex toy that is bound to be of great use?

Know What You Want

The very first thing which you need to do is first of all try and know what you want. Different people have different kinds of expectations and desires. You must perceive things in the right manner.

You should be willing to explore your inner realm and know the kind of fun and pleasure you are seeking. When you are willing to explore these specifics and you have a clearer picture of what you want, it would be much easier to buy the best sex toys.

Even if you are a little clueless; try to think of the kind of pleasure which appeals the most to you. If it is a deep orgasm that pleases you the most, you are in the mood for a vibrator. Similarly, if you are looking to explore the very insides of your vagina, you should settle for a dildo.

So, you have to truly explore your inner desires because buying that which you crave for seems like the right method to pick.

The Material

You cannot buy just about anything; the type of materials which they are made of assumes paramount importance. There are sex toys which you will be inserted inside your body. The last thing you want is to contract some kind of infection because you were too careless to check if the material was good enough.

So, one of the most important things to bear in mind when looking for the best sex toy is to check out the material they are made of and the quality standards they adhere to.

Mostly, it has been seen that metal, glass sex toys, and even silicone are some of the best choices at hand because they are non-porous. This ensures that they can be easily cleaned. At the same time, it also infers that there won't be any kind of rubber or bacterial infection with repeated use. So, both rubber and jelly are not advisable especially for the kind of sex toys which are pushed inside the genitals.

Battery Issues

There are two main categories of sex toys- rechargeable and battery-operated ones.

You need to decide the kind you want to opt for as this will have some impact on the ease of use which it will offer. If you go for rechargeable ones, they are likely to be environmentally friendly and at the same time, it is likely to be compatible with USB socket chargers. However, if you are mindful of the budget factor, you need to key in the fact that these are mostly expensive.

At the same time, if you choose battery-operated toys, they are also going to deliver the same level of performance. However, think of a situation wherein you are in between a sex session and using the toy to the fullest and the battery dies down. It could be such a massive dampener. So, the smarter thing to do in such cases is to go for rechargeable ones or always maintain a healthy stock of batteries so that the mood doesn't end up being spoiled.

The Noise Factor

Some of the sex toys like vibrators and even dildo make a great deal of noise. Now, if you are the kind who likes to have a little fun with sex toys in public places or even office, it becomes very important that you choose the ones which are discreet enough to keep the voice down.

The last thing you want is to let the whole office know that you are sneaking up and trying your hands at some odd sex job. So, check out the details of how much noise a sex toy would make and then decide accordingly as to what seems to be an apt choice for you. Some couples, on the other hand, use sex toys exclusively for the sake of turning themselves on at night. They might like a little noise to spice things up and if it can help them cut down the price, it doesn't hurt either.

So, find your priorities and choose accordingly.

The Utility

Another important factor which you should weigh when you are out buying sex toys is the kind of utility which they have. Whether you are looking for a massager, a vibrator, a cock ring, a dildo or anything else should be your final call. There is no dearth of variety as far as sex toys are concerned. This is why you have to meticulously go through the different options and then judge which toy seems like the thing you would like to try.

Once you are clear about the details, it should be easier for you to pick the right one. The idea here should be to step out of your comfort zone and experiment with something new and dynamic. When you do so, it is sure to ring in the right kind of response for you.

When you step out of your comfort zone to try something different, you might get hooked to the whole experience and end up falling it. So, there is so much to experience and explore the world of sex toys.

The Reviews

Even when you are going out to buy something as simple as a sex toy, we consider it a holy duty to go through the reviews. This is important because you do not want to invest in the cheap quality of sex toys which may not last long or lead to secondary infections. This is the reason; you should methodically check the review, inspect the details and come to the right conclusion regarding which of the toys seems to be the right one to pick.

Discreet Buying

Some of us are skeptical of heading to the sex store as we tend to judge ourselves for our choices. While we strictly believe that there is absolutely nothing to be ashamed of when it comes to buying sex toys, the underlying idea is to opt for online stores if you are not comfortable with the whole idea of going to sex stores.

However, when you choose to buy online, you need to ensure that you are sticking to the right stores and make sure that the packaging is done in a discreet way and doesn't come with big labels describing what is inside.

So, based on your personal choice, you have the option to pick whatever seems to be apt for you. Make sure to use all of the above points and you would then be in the best position to judge which tee seems to be perfect for bedroom game sessions.

The Toys For Men

Now, we are going to talk about some of the top sex toys for men which can help them explore their sexual depth and enjoy the sex to the fullest as well. This cannot be hailed as the ultimate list, because the definition of best toys is going to be very subjective. What appeals to you might not appeal to someone else's regardless, based on the general opinion, we have come up with this list which is likely to be a good pick for men.

1. The flashlights masturbator

This is handy and a perfect travel companion for those who love to masturbate. It is made of good quality materials and mimics the real act. The soft flesh at the top gives you the real feel and the design is ergonomic enough to help you have a good time.

A great choice and very popular among men who love to masturbate and relish the whole experience.

2. Autoblow artificial intelligence

Those of you who have a thing for blowjobs but haven't been lucky in this department can make a shift with this intimate product. It is a third-generation masturbation device that has been so designed that it gives you the same stimulation as the one you get whole having oral sex.

Not only this, it comes with an additional edging function too which can help you improve how long you last. The best thing is that it can fit any size of the penis; be it too small or large!

3. The Kiiroo TITAN

This is for those who want to experience life-shattering orgasms. This powerful device comes packed with several bursting bullets that shoot a vibration of their own and they make sure that each of them targets the right zone which has to be stimulated. It is best for those who are on the lookout for something kinky which could drive them to the very edge and help them experience the sheer pleasure of the ultimate climax.

So, these are the top picks within it comes to sex toys for men. Now, we are going to focus on toys to please the ladies too.

Sex Toys For Women

Now that we are done with objects to ease men, it is time for the ladies. Let us see some of the very best sex toys which women can use to give them the coveted world-shattering orgasms of all time.

1. We-vibe nova

This ultimate vibrator comes with a super flexible arm which is designed to bend in your body and give a deep thrust. The design is so ergonomic that you are sure to have your clitoris stimulated by it and your body will soon reach the ultimate level of deep satisfaction.

2. Eva 2 by Dame

If you are the kind of woman who likes to have both the clitoris and vagina stimulated all at once, we want you to opt for this magical toy. This sex toy comes with tiny little arms that will easily glide into your labia and the whole of the toy would sit smugly on the clitoris. The best thing is when your partner penetrates you on top of this or you conjoin it with a dildo, the orgasm is going to shatter your insides and outside and give you the kind of climax you have only seen in movies (porn ones that too!)

3. Gem by unbound

Glass dildos have become a massive rage these days and it shows how much women are looking to experiment with their body for the sake of enjoying the good times. This dildo is hard, inflexible and 100% safe. As it can be cleaned easily, it means that you won't contract infection easily. Also, it has been so designed that it can directly hit your G spot.

4. Sona Cruise by Lelo

If you are looking to venture into a deeper territory and want to opt for a new range of sex toys, this is the new option to look out for. They do not simply vibrate to give you the feel. These toys have been designed to emit sonic waves inside the system. This, in turn, sends pulses throughout the vagina and when it so happens, it ends up meticulously stimulating the clitoris.

A lot of people who have used this toy think that they could get a bone-chilling orgasm in a matter of a few seconds. So, if you want an out of the box experience, we thoroughly recommend you try this out.

5. Ora 2 by Lelo

If oral sex is something which turns you on and you are on the lookout for one of the perfect pieces, the smart gadget which you need to own has to be Ora 2. This is a smartly designed sex toy that is covered with soft silicone. When you feel it rotate, you will feel like your partner's tongue is giving you the steamiest oral sex on your clitoris.

No doubt, the kind of orgasms you will feel is sure to rock your world.

So, these are without a doubt some of the top picks as far as sex toys are concerned. The underlying idea is to ensure that you both end up enjoying the experience and live it to the fullest.

Fantasies for Couples

Our indulgence is something we are committed to and able to share with others. Seduction. Seduction. Mastery. Amazingly. An apparatus, atmosphere, or guidance that renders you attractive and inspires passion. Each shift is exciting to watch your wife. Become a sex toy of his or her own. Taste something different that you wanted to try always — with spectacular success. We are prepared for a beautifully hedonistic, romantic feast as we gorge on one another the tempting treats of sexual fantasy.

You can be swept from Kansas to Oz when you and you enjoy uncorking a magic bottle that holds your sexual fantasies. Sexual facts could render your usually great sex life spectacular, from an imagination flushed over during the lovemaking to a costumed role-playing game. Phantasies not only sizzle your mutual sex life, but they also bring your confidentiality to the next stage, expand communication lines, and enhance your senses. Fantasies are packed of suspense, excitement, risk, happiness, and love. And you can post them beautifully.

Are you constructing a Fantasy scenario If you imagine a particularly hot sexual position, maybe a twist or two, like making it public or seeing beautiful strangers? Do you become activated? Even if the elegance of dreams focused on imagined experiences does not reveal their potential of suspense — no makeup or different colors of lifestyle.

Fantasy simulations may take the idea "secret handwork" and provide it with a context— such as a theatre for films, a bar, an office, or a ride. Take the imagination and the fake handwork at the movie theater is from the alien seated next to you; it is from a waiter in the diner, and it's from someone at the workplace who wants the job you recruit. And you're turned into role-playing quickly if you attach costumes and props, clearly defined tasks, a plot with a start, the halfway point, and a conclusion.

Specific dream possibilities come in infinite variations. I suggest that you use your imagination and anticipation as a barometer to decide what will work best for you— you don't use your intellect. Combine fantasy elements that both trigger and tend to combine: a sex act, a piece of clothing, a location, a difficulty.

You and your friend were able to participate fairly— e.g., 69 behind a truck. Or you might call one-shots, run the show, enjoy the ride with the other one (or be "required" to join).

Here are some tips for launching you. You may draw up your imagination list of things that are cold and unsettling. You or your partner can select "yes," "no" or "maybe" next to each object to get a clear idea of what you would want to be playing with or to copy the lists below.

Sex Activities Masturbation of the penis, the mouth ejaculation, female ejaculation, genital penetration, pants, threesomes, two men, many spouses, sex toys, male receptive anal penetration, female receptive anal penetration, different roles, for example, doggie, being a core of the sex

None(nude), hangers, lingerie, men's clothes, neckties, briefs jumper, pants, boots, shoes, socks, fabric, elastic, latex, cotton, bandages, neck, wedges, linen, clothesline, frames, ribbons, bows in head, pigtails, bottles, skirts, formal dresses, tiaras, looking things including wedding coats, slippers, baths

Places and predictions Household (kitchens, offices, closets for the furniture, showers and toilets), vehicles, workshop, bike, fireplaces, barns, woodsheds, lake, pubs, aisles, dungeon, sex party and poolside, watching porn, especially sex act) Places and pillows, beaches, restaurants, bars (in a park)

Have you ever seen anything on these lists? A recollection spark? Well known sound? You may pick what things you want to render possible in the realm of imagination and work better. Most partners are more involved in playing with threesomes by imagining that there is a third partner in bed (with your most motivated dirty talk in fantasy) than by trying to find a right third partner. So bringing your husband to an imagined dog house in your bathroom is much better than chaining him back into your courtyard. In endless variations, you could mix imagined and specific circumstances, characters, and objects to optimize fantasy scenarios that enable you.

Face, or in reality?

How "true" it is to you to create your dream. When it comes to fantasy playing in your marriage, you have many choices. You can: • Hold your thoughts to yourself, enjoy them while coupling, and enjoy them for masturbation.

- Share your ideas and scenes during intercourse with one another by talking.
- Admit a dream you want to try— this may spark hot sex— even if the fantasy stays in the discussion.
- Talk about your ideas freely together and think about how you want to make them more practical.
- Build the situation in which the imaginations are realized.

Successful fantasy games need to take careful account of the situation, the pacing, and the physical and emotional comfort. This needs common sense, particularly. Facing it, the idea of playing a female employee who has been captured by a fantastic police officer— and hauled in handcuffed for a glamorous afternoon at the jail— might sound attractive, but it isn't enjoyable for anyone to get arrested.

For every fantasy that you make, from the fun wearing of slippers under a commercial suit to the duty of your boyfriend to have sex with a biker gang in a gas station. Accept both comfort and security criteria and mutually determine how far you want to push the creativity. The treats under his clothes may be sweet, but he might jeopardize his urinal behavior— or make his stall all day and feel uncomfortable rather than attractive. Or it could be part of your dream to feel uncomfortable: a quiet embarrassment that you don't have to provide for yourself. You won't have to worry — but you won't know how far in the creative mind, and what the boundaries will be to ruin the fun. You won't feel embarrassment. Likewise, the notion of "driving" your wife into sex can satisfy, but it can respond quite adversely to being bound, pulled around, or taken by surprise. On the other side, he can sincerely crave all this and worry that you don't go far enough.

A famous pornographic author, one of my closest friends, shocked me when I said to her about this novel. I had a confession. She was thrilled to hear that people want to live out their dream have a tool and needed it to be around for her when she offered almost anything almost a decade ago to have her husband spank her. "I had to be spanished still. But it took me two years to raise and tell my courage — and he was murdered! Another year I lived with him, and I felt depressed. She was too angry when I confronted my first husband because she thought it was' degrading' to girls, and he would never do so in the millions of years, and when she decided to be spanked, I assured him that it was the reverse. He went to my house about a week ago and purchased a hard backed comb, although he was always reluctant to take it, although I feel that's most of the time because he didn't know why. You may have the courage to ask for what you want, but it doesn't mean that you are fulfilled with excitement, or that, if you are, your partner has the knowledge and the ability to perform your wishes as you wants. Opening up can be terrifying, and even more disturbing is being greeted with fear, disappointment, and disgust. You will want to start learning how to communicate with each other and seek suggestions for starting the conversation.

Whether this is a lighthearted sex game or the unveiling of your most dark erotic dreams, imagination communication will bring you closer. You will figure out the most erotic secret desires of each other. Like excited teenagers on their first day, you are on a sexual adventure that takes you far away from your old sexual routines.

Your willingness to try (or at least discuss) new things gives rise to optimism. This is perfect for the friendship you have with each other. Our imaginations emerge from our deepest parts. We welcome someone else into our most private world once we reveal them. Emotionally exposed, it's simple. You have to trust your partner to refrain from assessing your skill, quality, and even more scarce imagination.

While such concerns can primarily be discussed by their talks, it becomes possible to increase confidence and to maintain this optimism over time. Not all will feel vulnerable to posting or dream screening. Some are empowered; many feel free to express themselves emotionally at last, and many more love the oral pleasure of speaking out loud about their wretched fantasies. If you let your desires go crazy, it cannot just make your sexual relationship intense, vibrant, and alive.

Most people find affection incredibly hot. Couples in long-term ties also find that incorporating dreams and role-plays to their physical practice opens up a whole new realm of sexual satisfaction, creates deep connections, and returns their vitality into the good old days of socialization and trial. You could set off some pretty powerful sexual chimes if you and your partner experiment through illusions as you would with a new sex toy.

Know your Lover's Fantasies

Getting to know your lover's imaginations It is as easy — and maybe like wrecking your lover's motors— to figure out what gets your lover going. You will want to read the whole chapter before you go to search for sexual gold when you frequently speak about gender, but sex is not a standard subject for you. Tell your friend what their dreams are, talk to them about some of your expectations, and see at the sparks fly. Or you can mention and share five sexual fantasies you are involved in. If you're a little tentative, but you can say that you're ready for something new, try to find out what they're involved in — a film scene of them catching a breath, a stuffy erotic novel on the

nightstand — and ask them in a provocative manner
what they like.

You will start to prepare your scene once you have a
fantasy subject in mind. First of all, decide what the
creativity is and to whom it refers. Is it your fantasy,
your partner, or both? Is it your creativity? You
already have all the dream elements in your mind if it
is yours, and you have only to give details to your
friend. See the first section of your fantasy thoughts if
your concepts are too sketchy to put into words— I
advise you to read them together. Choose a sex
activity, a costume, a pose like dominate and
submissive or tell your partner what the dream is.
Once you know who needs to do what, determine how
particular this situation is. You can remain in the
realm of imagination, view scenes in adult films, and
read each other's romantic stories, which represent
your fantasies. In this way, the mind is a vicarious
thrill, unbelievably hot and perfect for anxious
couples. This is a great experience. You also get the
pleasure from your sweetheart dream, or the comfort
of seeing your face seeing (or reading) your number
one switch.

You may go further with your fantasies and take a hot talk to sex, where the behavior of imagination in depth is represented by one participant. When you go about your daily sexual practice, you're getting contextual narrative.

You don't have to talk like a diva, a sexy porn star, to reflect your sex fantasies. Remember that the meaning of your vocabulary will be the subject of your lustful audience, not your language inflection or voice quality. Enable yourself to fall into the tale and feel free to fill in the air; it's a motor mouth that is for you.

Do you not know what to say? What to say? Accurately describe in as much detail as possible what you do or what your friend does. Let your definitions of sex bloom into a scenario you know you're going to like. For, e.g., when you sat on his face and strove his cock at the same time, describe the scene as if two of you were doing these things to him. That's — threesome dream moment!

Sexy surprises Quick seductions and mutually crafted dreams are among the most exquisite pleasures of life; however, they shock you with something you feel they would like for you to do. Be sure your partner understands something is imminent. Take care that you are not tired, have a rough day, or want to shave before you see. Prepare for a pleasant surprise ahead. Buy, get buttons, wear the right gear.

Surprise your friend for a sweet sexual surprise like an aphrodisiac or full-body erotic massage or read a fun tale (possibly one with your favorite).

- Stick a note telling them what they'd like to do together. So do it. So do it.
- Let your bags in your pockets, send them a letter with directions, leave an erotic image where they locate them, or bookmark an erotic novel, which you'd like them to learn.
- Stun you and execute one of your dream sex acts (like anal sex).
- Once you come home with a beautiful dress, welcome your companion once you realize that they like it and plan it for you to be turned into.
- You may be in a suit, a schoolgirl costume, wash in the bathroom, "take" the shower (or

watch porn, read a filthy novel, or what you shouldn't be doing).

- Transform your features in a sexy way, use romantic panties, and shaving your genitals. Try going out and tell your partner at dinner on a date that does not wear underwear.

The Sexual Buffet Decline takes many forms, but it may be the most thrilling and sensual dining encounters to give your lover a taste. Drizzle onto any part of the body that asks to be licked cocoa syrup, honey, and strawberry sipped and slathered creams. Nibble on the fruit you put on your skin, slip a delicious bug over your genitals and consume it in full view. Place your partner's meal on the boiling, excited torso (especially finger food such as sushi) and eat your sweet fill.

Make sure that your vagina does not contain sweets and that your diet is not analyzed (ever).

When you talk to your friend, Erotic thoughts will grow as quickly as you want to create a shared fantasy— as long as you wish. You could press emotionally, or share a lot of the same desires with your friend. And what you want, you must ask. A mixed response may be given — part interest, part terror. Some people are reluctant to even think about dreams, and some may be refused.

In any scenario, one of you wants to come up with an idea together — easy if you frequently chat about gender in your marriage, overwhelming when you never. In any case, it can seem daunting to tell your partner that you want to try something new— and if the dream makes you uncomfortable, this is an underestimation. Yes, it is sometimes also difficult to think about talking about sex!

If you have something that is known and tested about gender that you think can make your partner feel insecure, too, ask him or her that you want something to improve. This is particularly true of your sexual fantasy before you encountered your current partner. It requires quite a lot of grit to speak up and ask for something you want, but also to know more about what your partner enjoys or dislikes. And you can get what you want!

Until you do something, put yourself in the shoes of your partner: If you're still typically not talking about sex and then one of you needs to, it could start to get angry. If you had personal secrets all along, your partner would wonder. Your discovery of this romantic treasure trove will most definitely also give your partner the chance to tell you about sex.

Consider how you can make the subject feel safe for yourself: do you feel like watching a film that looks like your dream and reflecting on it after the show? Or do you think that you would be more comfortable waiting for your companion to get romantic and then tell you what they think of fantasy trading? You can also try to say that you want to reveal a fantasy—sex — and not have to respond instantly. Ask them that you can resolve things later; it allows you all the time to let the thought settle down.

Find ways to encourage your friend to listen to you. Tell them to suspend judgment before you realize how much fun you expect both of you will have — and how necessary their presence is for you. Make sure you tell him or her to be incredibly sexy and not to speak until you feel confident that you can share your deepest wishes. The partner has to know that they are the show's highlight–and that you can get stronger than you ever were. The main thing to consider in preparation is how you can help your partner feel comfortable. Mentally rehearse, once you have a discussion, what you want to convey. Talk about how your companion will respond, so you are prepared to take whatever direction the argument can go.

The partner may not want the erotic dream to be checked for a variety of reasons. Or you may wish to your companion to make you happy, but don't know what to do. The knowledge of these issues will help to talk constructively about the uncertainty of your friend, how to resolve doubts that can prevent one of you, and what to do if one person feels all right about the other.

It may create powerful feelings if your partner desires to physically attempt something that you are fearful of, unclear, or spiritual. The application of any new sexual activity to a marriage can sound like a case of making or breaking, and sometimes it is. Asking you to try forms of sexual intimacy can render your interaction more successful or can pose so many issues that the ship rolls — a little too much often. Fantasy will reach you at the heart if someone feels unsafe, unaware of the intentions of his companion, and deeply uncomfortable. This is particularly true in the case of deprivation, anxiety, gender, age, and violent fantasies.

You may be concerned that somewhere inside a wrong person, a person who "deserves" something harmful— or worse, you would like your dream to be real if your sexual fantasy simultaneously causes you uncomfortable and ridicule you (or, confusingly, excites you) at the moment. Fantasies of rape and incest are not rare but extremely disturbing. Such dreams are just that–illusions–and thus, they live in the realm of imagination or the security of fiction interacting with anyone you know.

Only imagination implies you don't want to see it put into effect.

Up to play? Are you armed for play?

You are suitable at playing now! Fantasies of natural sex acts can be performed when you're always prepared and wherever you want, with specific scenarios. Make sure you have protection. Home is the perfect place to play your game, so virtual sex partners will meet you with a little fancy talk and creativity to change the time and position you want, and you are free to use sex toys, fetish, and accessories to add to your enjoyment.

Take the time when both of you can be irritated and rest, turn off your mobile, make sure your roommates are genuinely home and give the children to a sitter. Make sure you search for products and items like a dog collar, whipped charcoal, full-length mirror, massage oil. Have your papers prepared beforehand or, if you are heading to the house of your wife, take your therapies. (Don't neglect your unholy imagination!). Above all, give a sense of sexual adventure and comedy as vision is just that — play.

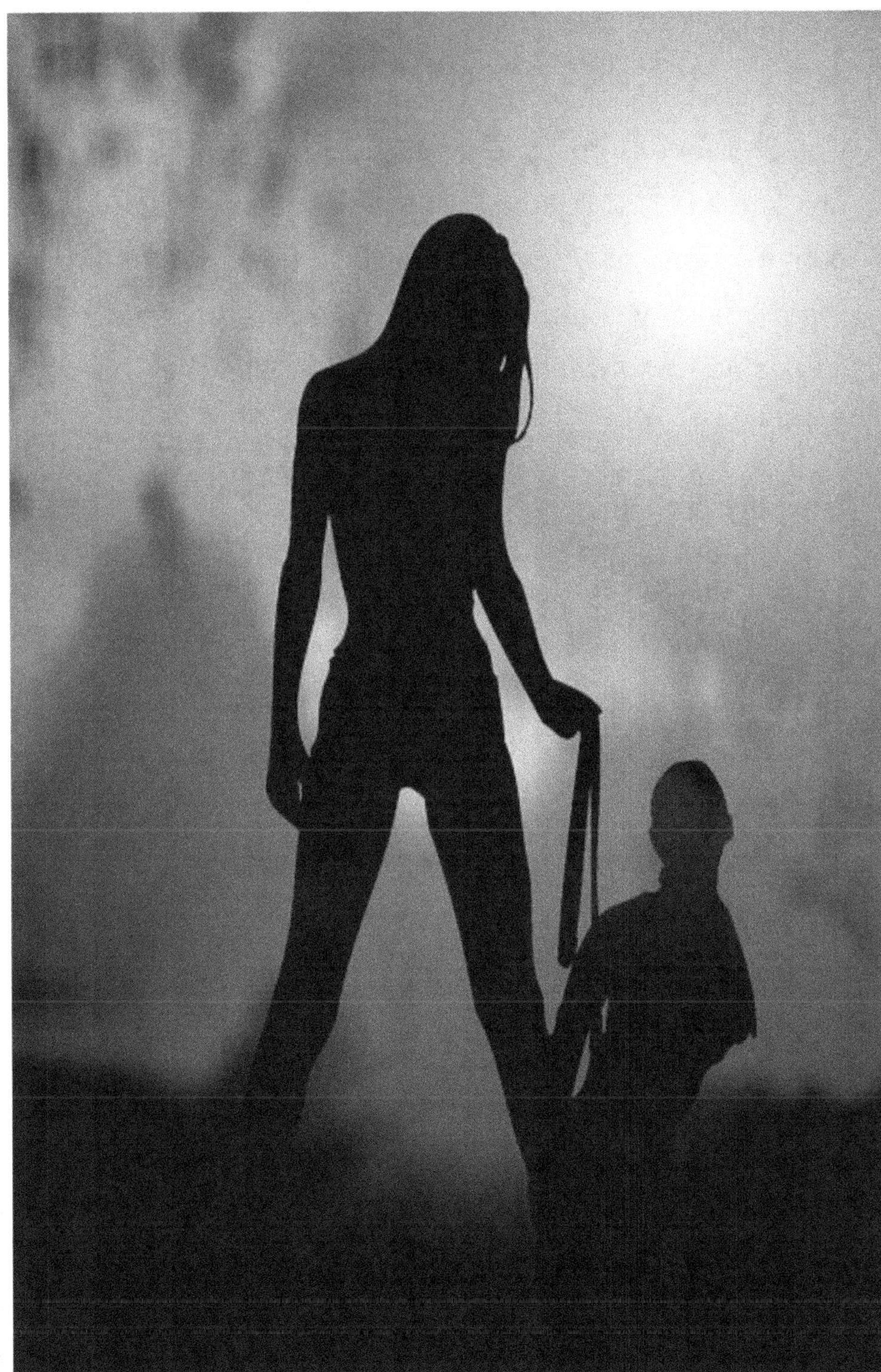

Chapter 5 Submissive Mindset

Not everyone is going to agree with how submissives are trained. But, it is between the submissive and her dominant and how they are going to go about getting the proper training for the submissive so that she or he is able to do what is necessary to make the dominant happy.

Human psychology

There is part of the human psychology that is being shaped when you are working to train a submissive. The people that you are around every day are being trained even if we do not do it on purpose so that decisions are made in such a way that the result that is delivered is what is wanted. This is what submissive training is going to do because as a dominant, they are going to spend time with their submissive.

When you go through submissive training, you are going to be having your behavior changed to match what ways that the dominant wants and get rid of or discourage those that they do not want. With patience, the way that a person acts can be completely changed so that they are someone that your dominant wants to be around twenty-four seven. However, it is crucial to make sure that both parties consent to what is happening! This is imperative when it comes to submissive training because this is the ultimate power exchange due to the fact that a dominant is getting into the submissive's mind and molding it to how they want it.

Training nowadays is not as bad as it used to be. In the old days, submissives were beaten to get the behavior out of them that they do not want. Now, it is done more subtly such as a sigh or a facial expression. This does not just happen in a dominant-submissive relationship; it also occurs in vanilla relationships.

Kink therapy

For dominants and submissives alike, the power exchange can be incredibly therapeutic. For a submissive, it is because they do not have to worry about their everyday problems. They are able to go to a different place and be someone that they are not in their daily lives.

Three aims for a submissive

As a submissive, there are three goals that you are going to want to get out of their training in being a good submissive.

1.   Behavior development: as a submissive, you are going to want to get rid of any behavior that your dominant does not like. The faster that you get this done, the better your relationship is going to be. It will be hard to change behaviors that you have done for most of your life, but it can be done.

When going through the act of training, you need to make sure that you are being trained by a person who is qualified in the skills that your dominant is wanting. Some schools are going to be able to train a submissive that are going to teach a submissive all of the techniques that are desired by a dominant. Some of these qualities are:

- Interpersonal skills
- Management of a household
- Event coordination
- Personal attendance
- Organization and communication for business

- Sexual service

Dominant's personal preferences

You are going to want to be trained to your dominant's personal needs and preferences. Not every dominant is the same just as not every submissive is the same. Instead of just sending them to a school to learn the most basic of submissive skills, a dominant may take it a step further and send their submissive to a yoga class in order to improve flexibility and more.

Some other things that a dominant may want their submissive to know are:

- food preparation
- specific rules for specific situations and the consequences for breaking those rules
- schedules for work and personal life
- fetishes that are preferred by the dominant
- and how to do the proper massage without harming their dominant

Personal goals

Even as a submissive you do not ever want to quit growing. You are going to want to set goals that are going to help you grow and become a better person as well as a submissive. For example, if you are not happy with how you look, then you can enforce a diet to make sure that you can get to how you want to look and your dominant should assist with that. Or, talk to your dominant about making space and time for you to do a hobby that keeps you centered so that you do not act out.

A submissive's role

Every person has a different desire to be a submissive. There are four different reasons as to why a person may become a submissive.

- Selflessness: they want to please someone else and do not necessarily want anything in return.
- Active service: a submissive that participates in active service means that they are doing things for others such as cooking or

managing a schedule if that is what is asked of them.

- Independence: being a submissive does offer a bit of freedom because you do not necessarily have to deal with everything on your own. There is someone there that is going to assist you in making sure that things are taken care of. To the degree that they go in supporting is going to be between the dominant and the submissive.

- Passive service: if something brings pleasure to someone else and it involves them, then the submissive will do it. So, if flogging the submissive brings pleasure to her dominant, then she will allow for it to happen.

Before you can figure out what kind of submissive you are, you are going to need to make sure that you are compatible in a dominant-submissive relationship and that your relationship is going to be a vigorous and healthy relationship that goes in a positive direction. It will also depend on the amount of training that you are going to require to make sure that you are doing what your dominant is desiring.

Of course, adopting a submissive lifestyle should not be done lightly but the topic should be allowed time to develop and ferment, and each member of the partnership should be willing to discuss what a sub/dom relationship means to them. If they are at odds, then rather than enhancing the relationship, it could considerably detract from it. If you agree to play the submissive to your partner's dominant, then you must ensure that you both have the right mindset. If you like the idea of being a submissive, but then baulk at the ideas your partner suggests, then you must work on acquiring the right mindset. This can take time but can always be achieved should you be willing to work on gaining the right attitude.

For instance, if your partner wants you to let him take the dominant role across the board, but you are used to making joint decisions, you must be willing to release your possession of control and give it up to your partner. Training might be done by the traditional spanking, which can be pleasurable to both parties. Not to put too fine a point on it, it could be compared to training Pavlov's dogs. You might come to expect being spanked when you know you are not being subservient but may submit because it is pleasurable. However, you may not always be in the mood to be spanked so you will try your best not to create a situation than warrants a spanking.

It is of no use carrying a resentful attitude around at being punished for stepping outside the boundaries or feeling that your partner is over demanding. Before committing to this lifestyle, you must discuss at some length what you want your relationship to be and how far you might be prepared to expand the boundaries of that decision. You must welcome the training and want to be submissive because you know that is what would please your partner.

If he insists that you cook his meals a certain way, you should do this from a standpoint of wanting to please him. He is your master and you should obey in much the same way as a dog does his master. You do it from a position of love and trust him to make the right decisions for you and the way your relationship develops. You must put your complete faith in that other person to make the right decisions for you. If you have this mindset, then you will thank him for doling out any punishment because you have willingly relinquished control to him in order that you can serve him properly and have the best relationship possible. He is in charge of shaping out the bond that a submissive needs to feel for their master.

If you have a high-powered job yourself, relinquishing power in your personal relationship to another person can be extremely liberating. If you have had to worry about bills in the past, that worry is now put upon the shoulders of the dominant. If you have grown tired of trying to think of meals to cook to please your dominant partner, he now takes that away from you and orders what he would prefer so that there is no deliberation required of you. You might also agree that he decides where you go on holiday or on who you mix with socially. How much pressure and tedium is you likely to be released from? Relax into a role of submission and enjoy the freedom that is likely to come with it.

Additionally, you must agree to leave your work in its proper place. If you have considerable rank and status at in the workplace, leave it where it belongs. Do not bring it into the home when you are trying to adopt a persona of being a submissive because it just will not work. Relax into the moment and ruminate about what you want to achieve, meditating if that helps. Leaving your work at work is a good practice to adopt in any circumstances so you are likely to benefit health-wise as your stress levels drops, perhaps lowering the threat of high blood pressure you've been exposing yourself to.

Sexually, it can be an exhilarating adventure. You must do as you are told and being ordered to perform a sexual act on or for your partner can be incredibly erotic. When your partner truly possesses you sexually, it can result in a huge turn-on.

If you should find yourself struggling to adopt this mindset, ask your partner if you can talk about it in more depth. Try to explore why you feel the way you do and where those feelings come from. Exploring the reasons why you feel as you do can often release pent up worries and fears and allows you to excavate deeply within yourself and expel negative and useless thoughts and feelings.

Meditation can often help you sort the wheat from the chaff and lead you down the path that is truly for you. If you have never tried meditation, it can be extremely illuminating. All it requires of you is that you find a quiet place, preferably where you are alone and will not be disturbed. Keep your feel flat on the ground and your back straight. Breathe in to the count of seven and out to the count of nine and as you do so become aware of your breathing. Clear your mind of all things, which are fighting for dominance in your brain and relax. If thoughts persist acknowledge them and decide to deal with them at a later time. Now is your time. After a period, such as this, you may well find that your thoughts become much more lucid. Arguments that jostled for dominance now will find some semblance that you recognize as being rational and lead you to where you want to be. It can be a confusing time when you are struggling with your sexuality on any level and this is a very useful technique to clear the clutter of what does not matter and is no longer relevant to who you are now.

For some, being totally submissive in all areas of their lives becomes totally natural and it is a simple return to the 1950s when women knew their place. This was possible because they were indoctrinated from all sides: parents, government, and the media. The economy was such that women were easily controlled and just as easily they believed that their place was in the home, tending the children and doing as their lord and masters bid.

The role of the submissive seems even to have been enshrined in law and seemed to indicate that women do not necessarily realize how much power they have and if used wisely, their feminine wiles can ensure that they achieve the perfect relationship. Men certainly seem to have done and found it necessary to make laws about women getting above their station thus allowing them to retain the power, which had evolved over centuries into their ownership. This is why it might be surprising to some how quickly the scales seem to be tipping and rebalancing the ratio of power in recent decades. It is no wonder that both genders are fraught when trying to find their place in a new world that they no longer recognize from that of their parents'.

However, historically at least, women have been more naturally caregivers and can take enjoyment from serving another. She might make sure that her Dom has eaten enough or that the food is cooked exactly to his liking. By the very fact that she cares about these things, when they are right means that she can derive pleasure and comfort from being able to please in all areas of their shared lives together. Although this is probably the case now, there are gently shifts away from it as the role of house husband becomes more acceptable and common on modern society.

Zoe Eckman, which was, encapsulated another angle of exploiting feminine prowess in a well-known quote: "An Angel in the Kitchen, a Lady in the Living Room, and a Whore in the Bedroom." This seems to imply that women are adept at managing several roles consecutively. If a man feels dominant and happy in that role, how much more likely is he likely to be to want to keep his little lady, who answers his every whim, completely and thoroughly happy in every respect?

It may be more difficult to attain the mindset now in a world of burgeoning equality between the genders, but it is still possible. If you commit to living out this lifestyle, the more you do it, the more natural it will become. It will edge out into other areas of your life perhaps without you even being aware it is doing so.

Others find it erotic to exploit their naughty side at intervals and adopt it solely for this reason. And why not? It does not have to be all encompassing. If you prefer to dip in and out of a sub/dom relationship and take only the sexual role-playing part, then that is fine too. It can still enhance your relationship. In fact, you may find it easier to take on the persona in part or parts rather than in entirety. But, as expressed above, you might find this expanding into other areas of your life imperceptibly.

If you feel comfortable with this and want it to spread into all areas of your life, you are lucky. If, on the other hand, you feel silly or foolish trying to settle into this role, then take it steadily and introduce it bit by bit. Ask yourself – and your partner – why you want to add it to your lives. Become comfortable talking about it and accept it as part of your natural lifestyle. In this way, your mindset will adjust to it more readily.

On the other hand, if you feel it is unnatural, you are unlikely to gain much pleasure from it. Do not agree to it if this is the case if it is only to give your partner pleasure. If you do this, you are likely to feel resentment at some point and it will have a contra effect on what you are trying to achieve. When you are trying to achieve the submissive mindset, try and block out thoughts that lead you away from it. Try and focus, perhaps counseling could help to get rid of controlling thoughts from your past?

Or, alternatively, at the other end of the scale, when you become more practiced and relaxed, it might be a physical movement from your dominant such as a smack on the bottom or just a look. You might find that sometimes it his easier than others to slip into a submissive mindset. On one day, you'll really be feeling it and enjoying it; on others, you can't seem to get it. On these days, play along. It is a little likes strengthening a muscle and the more you use it, the stronger it becomes.

When you're starting a new relationship, or even deciding to adopt it in an already established one, it will be necessary to be trained in the needs of your dominator. It can often prove useful to formalize this training, so you might agree that it should be written down so that you can become familiar with it and refer to it often. This list could even be used as a contract between two consenting parties and used as guidelines for the terms of your relationships. Not only does this help the submissive know what they must do to please their partner, it outlines the boundaries, which the sub has agreed they do not want to overstep. For instance, it might say that no leather belts or whips are to be used. Of course, as the relationship advances, the tolerance for pain might grow and it is always possible to revisit the contract and amend it accordingly.

The contract might include details about if there are to be any names allocated to the sub and dom. Some couples like to use Sir or Master while the sub might be called baby or doll. You might already have your own names that you prefer to use for each other. It should include instructions on each area your relationship covers. Does it only cover the sexual area, or does it stretch into the financial or domestic areas? Is it to be kept completely private or are you going to go public and preserve this relationship in front of others?

It can be general but might need to be adjusted as you get to feel your way around the relationship. If this is in an established relationship, then drawing a contract up can be very useful too. It allows the couple to discuss the terms of their relationship in detail, but it doesn't necessarily have to formal and serious; it can be light-hearted and fun – and incredibly sexy. Just talking about what you want to happen sexually might produce a sexy scenario – or two – when you decide to practice and live it out there and then and certainly serves to get you both in the right mindset. This can't be a bad thing as you are already enlivening your sex lives together. It can also re-enliven a marriage which has become stale and predictable and lead you back to times when you found sex highly exciting and looked forward to it rather than it being something to simply get through. It calls upon you both to be imaginative and creative and to consider in depth what sex means to you.

It's up to the both of you to decide how precise you want this contract to be. It might be so explicit that it includes things such as: Master to spank baby at 8 p.m. every Friday night and baby must be dressed in whatever Master wants and be prepared and waiting in the bedroom. It could then go onto say what she will be expected to do afterwards sexually. Alternatively, it might outline domestic duties and the way that the dom's coffee should be and when he should receive it. This is an entirely personal thing between two people and this can change with each new partner. Never assume that a sub's training is the same for every relationship because sexual preferences will be different for each person.

Needless to say, part of the fun is finding out what suits you both best and can be unbelievingly erotic in a new partnership and even more mind-blowing in an established one.

Vulnerability

Being a submissive takes a lot of courage due to the fact that you are exposing yourself to another human being. The scariest part does not know if they are going to take the information that you give them and use it against you or if they are going to protect it and use it to make your relationship better.

As you open yourself up to someone else, you are going to be telling them some of your darkest secrets and deepest desires. Things that you have not necessarily shared with anyone else. This vulnerability can be scary for anyone, however, having open lines of communication will aid in being able to talk to your Dom and expose yourself.

When it comes to the sexual aspect of being vulnerable, you are entrusting your dom with your safety and pleasure. Whenever you are in a scene, you are going to have a say in what happens, but for the most part, it is going to be in the hands of your master.

You are most likely going to be experiencing new things at the hands of your partner. The feeling of knowing that he is not going to hurt you (once you have established that trust) and the feeling of not knowing if you are going to enjoy what is going to happen can leave you feeling vulnerable as well. Especially in the event that you are not able to see what is going on.

There is a wide range of issues that can make you feel vulnerable, especially if you have been abused in some fashion in your past or if this is your first relationship. A real Dom is not going to take advantage of your vulnerability and they are not going to abuse you. In fact, a real dom is going to help nurture you and show you that you have no reason to feel vulnerable because they are there to protect you.

Being exposed sexually or at all can get in the way of your relationship with your dominant, but you have to believe that your dominant is going to take care of you. If you are still having issues with feeling vulnerable, that is when you need to open up a dialogue and speak to them about what you are feeling. Perhaps you are in need of further help than what they can provide for you. If that is the case, then they are going to help you heal and get past what is holding you back.

As was mentioned earlier, if this is your first serious relationship, then you are going to be more vulnerable due to the fact that you are not going to know what to expect. This is where a lot of doms may come in and attempt to take advantage of the fact you do not have much knowledge or any experience. You are going to have to watch out for these people because you are going to be a prime target for them.

Do your research and find someone who is willing to mentor you. There are always going to be vulnerabilities due to the fact that you are opening yourself up to someone else without knowing if they are going to use that knowledge for good or to harm you. But, if you have found the right dominant, then you are going to have someone who is going to take care of you and make you feel secure enough to push those things that make you feel vulnerable and blossom into a stronger person.

Vulnerability can have many meanings. While it can convey weakness, defenselessness and helplessness, it can also be interpreted as meaning openness and exposure. Unscrupulous people are likely to choose the first meanings and use your enthusiasm to co-operate sexually as levers for exploitation. However, genuine people will see it as a means of getting to know each other better. In fact, this is a perquisite for finding out about another person and getting closer to them, forming meaningful bonds. You are both allowing yourselves to be open with each other and share experiences and feelings. Revealing yourself to others can open you up for abuse and if you do not consider yourself naturally good at getting along with people and connecting with others, then you should proceed with the utmost of care.

If this is not a longstanding relationship, you must always be responsible for your own safety. As in any kind of sexual relationship, there are unscrupulous, even psychotic, people who enjoy hurting others for the sake of it. Agreeing to being placed into a vulnerable position, especially physically, is opening yourself up to potential danger, especially in new relationships but can also equally apply to established ones.

Always have a safe word, which you have agreed beforehand with your partner. Be aware that this should not be a run of the mill word but should be so unusual for the other person to stop in his tracks and react to. Make it quite clear to him that if he does not abide by your terms of keeping safe, then it is a no-go area. You need to have complete and utter faith that you are safe, or you will not be able to relax into the role and enjoy it for what is it. You should feel excited but unafraid.

You should also have some plan of escape should things get out of hand. Don't let someone you do not know very well tie you up in a totally isolated place where it would be impossible to attract attention and call for help. You should not allow yourself to be gagged by people who you are not completely sure of so that this does not become possible. Just because you are in a highly aroused state doesn't mean that common sense should fly out of the window.

The very nature of a sub/dom relationship is that one person should feel vulnerable/submissive. The relationship is allowing another person to take control of you so completely that you will feel in their power, i.e. vulnerable. But be careful not to confuse the feeling of vulnerability in a trusting and caring relationship to feeling so vulnerable that you feel frightened of what is going to happen and worry for your own safety. There is a difference and you should be able to distinguish which one you feel quite easily. If you are in any doubt about which emotion you are experiencing, ask him to stop. Even if he is in a highly aroused state, you should never feel afraid under any circumstances. You should be able to trust him that he will never overstep the mark and believe that you have the power to instantly stop anything that you do not want or welcome.

As any relationship develops, whether it is sexual or not, it should involve showing the other person your vulnerable side. It's about sharing things about yourself with them so that it is acceptable to show that you're human like them, not superhuman. It's intimacy in its truest form.

Do not think that vulnerability necessarily must be equated with weakness. It can be an indication of strength if you are willing to expose your emotions, fears, and aspirations to another person. You exchange your power and get to know the person much more thoroughly in this fashion because you are allowing them to see your hidden emotional parts, those parts you only show to people you trust, or want to trust in the future at the very least.

Be prepared: there will be times that you get hurt. To go through life expecting never to feel pain would be unrealistic. Lower your guard and let people see the real you. If you turn off that need to connect to others, your life is likely to be lonely. Showing your vulnerable side to people you wish to connect with opens up fresh avenues where you can relate on a number of levels. If you do this, and discover a mismatch, this might mean that you are not compatible, or it might mean you need to work on your relationship so that you become more compatible. Showing your vulnerability is perversely a very brave thing to do but it doesn't mean you expose yourself to danger at whim, so this course should be employed with commonsense and caution.

Showing your vulnerability does not entail telling everyone you meet every detail about yourself. You must use your own wise judgment that should be told what and when. Telling people your whole life story as soon as you meet means there is nothing left to find out about. Try and keep a little mystery so that others want to learn more about this fascinating new person that they've just met. If you were to reveal everything immediately people might perceive it as odd in any event. Think Forrest Gump here.

People must earn this honor because it is indeed an honor to have your deepest secrets and hopes and fears revealed to them. They should treat it as the treasure it is and respond in kind. That is when there is a true connection between two individuals. Don't be afraid of being the first to say, "I love you" when you enter a new relationship, but on the other hand don't be so ready to tell everyone you meet. You should know when it is time instinctively and outdated societal rules should not hold you back. Remember, it's a precious gift you can share with others. Treat it as such.

If you're vacillating about whether you should show your vulnerable side and agree to become a submissive, ask yourself what is the worst that could happen? Why do you feel afraid of showing your vulnerability? Is it a fear that if you show someone who you are, they will reject you and consider you unworthy of their affection? That is always a risk, but life tends to remain dull and boring if you are unprepared to take any risks at any point. Is the action about to become irreversible? Is it not something, which you could write up to experience and say, 'Well, I tried it but it's not for me'? Without some measure of vulnerability, you will never be able to develop relationships because they grow when people share things about themselves and that always has the potential to make a person vulnerable.

And don't try sharing personal things about yourself to get a shock reaction. Telling someone that you've had a breast removed on your first meeting might be considered as being highly irregular and off the board, not to mention being construed as needy. You are definitely not looking for a reaction to a 'poor me' persona. You are trying to reveal things that give you a connection to the other person, looking for things, which you have in common and resonate soundly with them.

By showing your partner that you can be vulnerable and that you are willing to try what he suggests, takes a courage that you may not be aware you possess. In fact, being vulnerable is a very necessary and vital part of your role as a submissive and vulnerability can be exercised and enjoyed.

Allowing your vulnerability to show through exposes how authentic you are. You are being yourself and not afraid to show others who you are. Presenting the real you, warts and all, gives others license to be themselves too and encourages a reciprocal honesty on their part. It engenders confidence because if you have shown someone who you truly are and confessed your fears and they still love you, there is nothing left to fear. They love you for who you are. In fact, you might expect that a vulnerable person is a dependent person who needs the affirmation of others to validate who they are. In fact, the opposite is true. To show your vulnerable side often indicates that you are self-confident. You are happy to be who you are and happy with the way your life is going.

Self-deprecation, however, can be attractive but it's all about degrees. If you constantly go around using the 'Poor me' tone, you are going to be perceived as a boor and a bore and people will start avoiding you like the plague because they fear you are too needy and will place unreasonable demands upon them. Not only is this not sexy, it is a total turn-off.

If you come across someone who has had multiple serious relationships or has turned into a serial bride or groom, there has to be something suspect there. If a person cannot be sure that they are capable of being part of a healthy relationship, then they should be willing to work on it and take some of the blame for things going bad repeatedly. If their relationships keep breaking up, this might be an indication that there is something wrong. It might indicate that they were not happy to show their vulnerability at all, or it could be that they became totally vulnerable and dependent on another person. If this is you or you recognize any of these patterns, be honest with yourself and start working on it. You have to be an active participant in changing your life for the better.

Being brave enough to be vulnerable also encourages someone to look after you and treat you properly. But this has to be coupled with respect for that person who has overcome the bad times in their lives and is now strong enough to share it with another person. They want you to be safe and never have to face misfortune again because they want to look after you. If you should come across someone who takes advantage of any vulnerability you show and abuses it, ditch them or at least tell them they have overstepped the mark and must agree to renegotiate the terms of your relationship.

Learn to use vulnerability to its full effect. It is a very powerful tool in your armament and you should never underestimate it. Showing your vulnerability might be as simple as relating stories of funny things, which have happened to you. Again, don't make a habit of this or you will just be perceived by others not as someone who is simply entertaining but as an idiot. Try to employ humor so that others can detect that you don't take yourself too seriously. If you can make someone laugh, they are more likely to sympathize with you when things go wrong.

Vulnerability is not about a Mills and Boon heroine swooning in her lover's arms – although of course it can be if that's your thing. In today's modern world, where the sexes burgeon for equality, it involves a woman who is sure of who she is, has the strength of character to survive, but has the strength to still reach out and say, this is the naked me and I need you to make me happy.

Showing your vulnerable side also requires that you are optimistic. If you find yourself always looking on the worst that could happen, you must learn to stop in your tracks. Try and evaluate what adverse implications an event happening could bring to bear on your life. Would you die? The answer is probably not. Bad experiences make us stronger – or at least they should do. Look back on your life now. What things stick out to you as most memorable? Is it the bad things or the good ones? It's okay if some bad things spring to mind, as long as you learned something from the experience and feel enlightened by them. A very real example, which comes obviously to mind, is childbirth. It can be horrendously painful but as a reward for the pain, at the end along comes one of the best prizes in life you can receive.

Hopefully, the bad times have been few and far between and the endless nights you've experienced in the past are gone and forgotten, or at least stored away so that they don't hurt anymore. Conversely, you should try your best to remember all the good times, including the best sexual experiences that you've had. Doing so, will make you a happier person who people will be likely to gravitate towards.

It's most the amazing thing when a person who is happy and brimming with confidence, always ready to help others, opens up and reveals something which they've rarely or never admitted to anyone else. What is being shared then is something, which is a very precious commodity. That person is revealing a very private and intimate part of themselves, which they might not trust with someone else. They are showing their vulnerability. Even though they may have been hurt so many times before, they are trusting you with information that has the potential to be used against them to do them harm. Treasure this. It truly is a gift worth having and means that you have made a very meaningful and intimate connection with another human being.

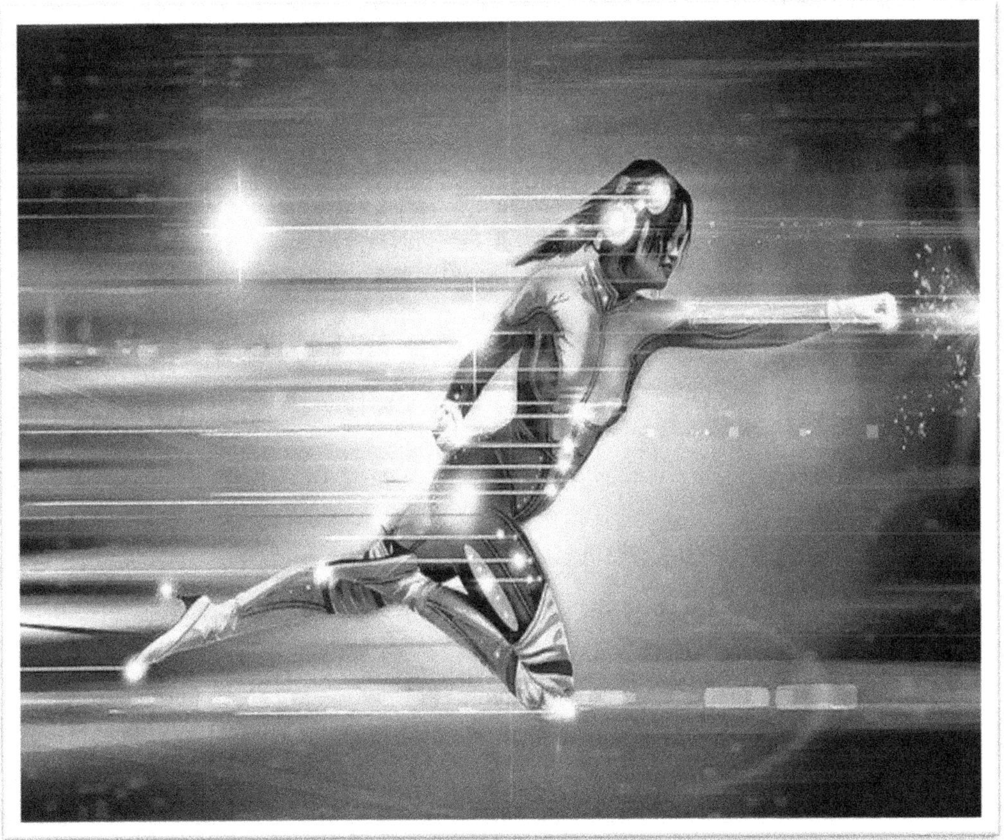

Chapter 6 Techniques For Stronger Erections

When you are engaging in an act of sex, the kind of erection which you get assumes gargantuan importance. Men are always very skeptical of the kind of erection they are getting. If they do not get a very strong boner, they may feel apprehensive about their sex performance.

When you are in the mood and actually turned on, it is natural for you to get a boner. But some men may not get very strong erections. In such cases, it becomes even more important to know the best techniques by which you can achieve it.

Why Some Men May Not Get Strong Erections?

There are several reasons as to why men get weak erections. We will shed light on some of them.

- Low blood flow: By far, the most common problem has to be limited blood flow to the penis. It is when the blood is pushed to the penis that it increases in size. So, if the blood flow is limited, it can lead to weak erections.

- Blood pressure problems: Those patients who tend to suffer from high blood pressure may have weaker erections.

- Cholesterol: Patients with high cholesterol too can have hardened arteries that in turn mean limited blood flow. This could lead to a weaker erection.

- Diabetes: Those people who are suffering from diabetes are much more likely to be patients of erectile dysfunction. Diabetes tends to have a direct impact on the penis and can also cause severe damage.

One of the pivotal things which you need to know is that there has to be ample blood flow to the penis when you are looking to get an erection. This is why foods that are good for the heart tend to have a direct impact on the quality of erection which you get. When your heart is healthy, your sex life too is likely to tick off in the right direction.

The Right MethodsTo Use

In this chapter, we are going to talk about different ways and methods which will come to your help when you are looking to get a bigger and stronger erection.

Always make it a point to opt for a mix and match of these tips and methods as it is sure to bring in the right results for you.

The Diet Sheet

Yes, once again, the food that you eat is of paramount importance when it comes to getting an erection. There is plenty of bad food which is not good for men who are looking to get a stronger erection. So, when you seem to be struggling with this problem, it is even more important to mind what you eat. Here, we are going to give you some important tips and suggestions with regard to your eating habits that will be of help.

The Good Food

A typical Mediterranean diet that is rich in fruits, vegetables, healthy fats, and even whole grains is likely to help men achieve stronger erection. You need to include plenty of fruits and vegetables in your diet. Also, nuts, olive oil, fish and related healthy products might do you a world of good.

Along with this, blueberries are known to be one of the favorite products which you have to eat. They are rich in anthocyanin which is an antioxidant. The presence of this antioxidant helps in cutting down the level of free radicals in the body. This in turn aids in better blood flow to the penis.

Further, food rich in B12 can also aid in better erectile health. Things like fermented soy-based tempeh and other vitamin-rich sources of food are sure to aid in improved health and better and stronger erection.

Not only this, leafy vegetables like spinach can also aid in improved testosterone levels. It is also rich in blood circulation.

While there are the details of the food that you need to eat, you also need to be mindful of the ones which you should skip.

The Bad Food

Eating fried food, processed ones, and fat-rich food might not be a good thing to do. These foods tend to lead to several problems which include heart ailment, diabetes, and blood pressure. Each of these problems has been linked to the possible cause of erectile dysfunction. So, by sticking to a bad diet, you may be creating a lot more problems for you.

The key is to always find the perfect balanced diet which is rich in minerals and nutrients and strict to it.

Alcohol And Smoking

There are a few lifestyle habits that are known to have a bad repercussion on your sex life. You should make it a point to limit both alcohol consumption and smoking tendency from your lifestyle.

There is plenty of research which has indicated that higher consumption of alcohol is known to have a direct impact on your sexual drive. While we are not asking you to completely get rid of it, it has been seen that heavier consumption of alcohol tends to be harmful to your sex drive. It could have severe negative repercussions and may even curb the desire to have sex. It is okay to drink in moderation, in fact, that might help you boost the sex drive. However, you need to know where to cross the line because overdoing it is sure to create all possible kinds of troubles.

Even when it comes to nicotine, the impact is long-lasting and severe. Cigarettes, vaporizers are known to have an adverse impact on your blood vessels.

When you take a puff of a cigarette, it cuts down the utility of nitric oxide. Nitric oxide is needed in the body because it aids in the smooth flow of blood. It is the presence of this compound in the body which helps in opening the blood vessels to facilitate easy movement. So, when the consumption of nicotine interferes with the utility of nitric oxide, you will find a reduced supply of blood. This, in turn, might lead to troubles like erectile dysfunction in the long run.

Along with this, there are also reports which hint that smoking tends to bring damage to the penile tissue in particular. This ends up impacting the elasticity of the penis adversely and consequently, it may not be able to stretch as much as it could otherwise.

Exercise

There are no two stories as to why exercise is absolutely crucial when it comes to enjoying the best of health perks. Be it getting stronger erections or enjoying a better sense of mental peace or staying agile all across the day, the benefits are there for each one of us to see and experience.

You can opt for an hour or aerobic exercise as this will help you keep your body on the move. Mostly, every logic boils down to improving the kind of blood circulation which you have. The erection is all about the rush of blood in the penis area.

In today's fast-paced corporate lifestyle wherein most people spend a large part of their day sitting on the chairs; you must invest in healthy exercises and even simple activities like walking. Even if you walk just 2 miles a day, you are likely to steer clear of the problems of erectile dysfunction. Walking too tends to open all the blood vessels and thereby permits the healthy flow of blood to all areas.

Sleep Cycles

We all know how important it is to get adequate hours of sleep. When you are sleeping regularly, your body tends to replenish and rejuvenate. It is not a surprise that men get several nocturnal erections stretching anywhere from three to five and possibly more. The duration of these erections could be as long as an hour as well.

Have you ever wondered as to what is the main aim of these erections and why do they occur when you are neither horny nor thinking of having sex? The answer is simple; the erections are mainly to help in recharging your penis. This helps in supplying the penis with a rich supply of oxygenated blood.

When you get multiple erections during the night, it will help in making your erectile tissue a lot more flexible and more elastic as well. So, there is no doubt that your sleep cycle and also the quality of sleep which you are getting assume paramount importance.

Do whatever it takes to get a good quality of sleep. You can make use of soothing music or even think of sleep-inducing activities. Make sure to wear comfortable clothes and have the best comfy mattress. Every step is going to make a difference.

Curb The Anxiety Regarding Your Penis Size

One of the terrible things which most men do is worry constantly about the size and quality of erection they are getting. What you need to clearly understand is that anxiety or worrying about the penis size is no way going to help your case. Rather, it is a perfect recipe to create many more problems for you.

This is why you have to first believe in yourself. Regardless of how small or big, your penis is, stop fussing about it. If you are not getting an erection, your focus should be on finding ways to fix the problem. Simply worrying about it is not going to sort the matter for you.

When you are anxious or stressed, it tends to increase the levels of the adrenaline hormone in the body. This hormone is known to constrict the blood vessels. Hence, there is scientific evidence to prove that anxiety and tension can prevent you from getting stronger erections. When you understand the utility of your action and you are willing to put in a wholehearted attempt for the sake of dealing with this stressful trouble of erectile dysfunction, you may be in a better place to handle it.

Handle Relationship Woes

Some people get a strong erection when they are masturbating but somehow when they are having sex with their partner, they fail to get a strong erection. If this is the case with you, it is time to handle your relationship woes. If you are not happy with your partner or there is some issue bothering the two of you; you must know how to handle it. Talk to each other out and sort the matter.

No relationship can continue for long if you do not feel the passion kick between the two of you. So for couples who are at loggerheads, they should try their best and do whatever it takes to iron out the differences and gap which is present between the two of you. Often, it is these little things which can help you come closer and this, in turn, might help you once again enjoy the sex.

Try New Things

Sometimes, sex gets boring and when it gets boring, you may not be in the mood for erection. Naturally, the penis tends to get erect when you feel a strong urge to have sex. So, this is why you should always make it a point to keep sex exciting, new, and fun.

This is the reason; we encourage you to try new things and ideas when you are looking to have sex. From picking the best of new positions to springing horny surprises, trying sex toys and even experimenting with different kinds of sex accessories might be a great way to push things to an altogether new level.

When you do so, it is likely to help you get better at the erection game eventually. There is no limit to the kind of fun and experiments you can have when you are trying to have sex. So, be willing to explore new realms and see what your partner feels when you are looking to have sex.

Battling Stress Woes

Last but not the least; you have to clearly understand that stress is one of the major reasons for this problem. Stress can arise because of several reasons and things. When you want to work on your body, you have to limit all levels of stress as much as you possibly can.

You can indulge in breathing, meditation, and yoga sessions and each of these are likely to help you deal with stress. When you do so, it will give you a better incentive to be happy. When people are happy and not constantly worrying, their mood is in an elevated sense and this, in turn, will help you have a better sex drive. Most people tend to look forward to sex when they are in a happy mood.

The Sex Positions

It is important to pitch in this extra point in the end. While we are not asking you to be extremely cautious when you are in the mood for sex but always remember not to get too forceful when having sex. Some positions wherein you thrust a bit too harshly can be harmful to your penis. The last thing you want is to realize that you end up hurting your penis and shriveling it simply because you were too overzealous. So, be experimental and try new positions for sex, but in the end, you need to understand the best ways to exercise caution when engaging in sex.

The focus should always be on attaining pleasure and not measuring how hard, vigorous, or fast you are. So, these are some of the things you need to keep in mind when you are looking to have stronger erections. You must pay heed to each of these aspects because problems like erectile dysfunction have the tendency to crumple your sexual life after all.

When you implement a mix of the above tips, we are hopeful that it will help you get stronger erections. If the problem persists, we recommend you to visit a specialist and consult him immediately. Erectile dysfunction is not a problem that should be taken lightly. There are herbal supplements and medicines which are available that can help you get stronger and larger ejections but what you need to know is that not all of them are safe. This is the reason, consulting a doctor is recommended before you do any of it.

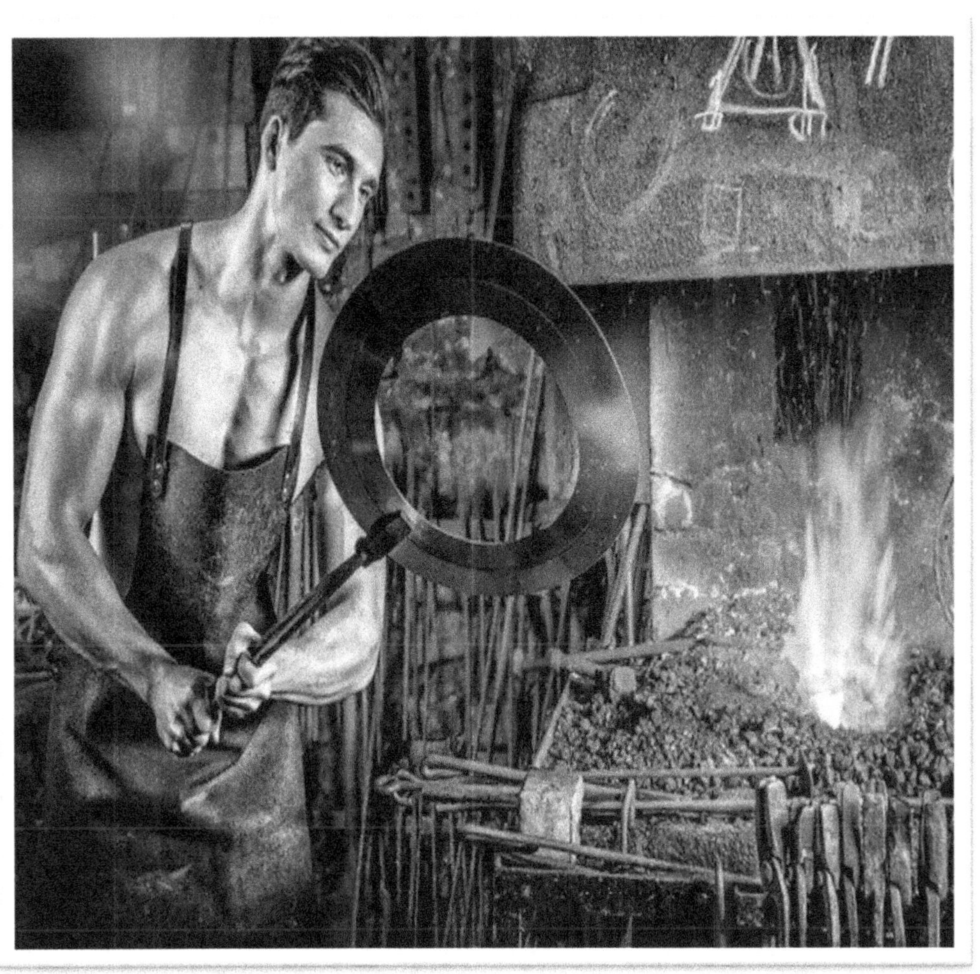

Chapter 7 Spicing Up Your Sex Life

Wake up. Go to work. Come home. Exercise. Eat. Have sex. Sleep. Repeat. We're creatures of habit and routine. While that's not necessarily a bad thing, it can put your sex life at risk of becoming dull, mundane, and well, just plain **boring.**

Overcoming the Boredom

As much as we may love our partners, it has to be said that boredom does happen. When it hits, some couples may be tempted to go astray when they feel emotionally and sexually bored. By nature, humans are attracted to change. We need variety now and then to keep things exciting. Even when venturing out of our comfort zones is not something we seek out actively, a little excitement that shakes things up once in a while can make us feel alive again. When everything becomes too routine, boredom inevitably follows.

We choose to make that commitment and get into long-term relationships for several good reasons. We want the emotional security that comes with it, we want the happiness and sense of belonging that comes from sharing a special bond with another. Yet, at the same time, by committing to one relationship, we are also limiting our option. Could it be fair to say that boredom was perhaps inevitable? We're living longer, enjoying greater leisure, and we've got higher emotional and sexual expectations from our partners. These and a lot of other factors today make it unlikely that couples who stay together for decades will **never** experience boredom together.

For many couples, particularly the ones who believe in romanticized versions of love and marriage, disappointment, hurt, and sadness quickly follow when they realize their partner may be boredom with their sex life. The electrifying passion they once felt begins to wane over time. The sex starts to get too routine and mechanical. Some people feel unhappy and grieve over the loss of that aspect of their sex life, while others may stray. But there are couples who do something else entirely. They find **new** ways of keeping the excitement alive in their relationship. Yes, breathing life back into an old relationship is absolutely possible, but it does require that the couple work together to get it done. To rekindle the excitement, couples need to surprise each other in new and unexpected ways. Not just physically, but emotionally too. Introduce new ideas in the bedroom, try new positions, use sex toys, maybe even venture outside the bedroom to find the cure of sexual boredom. How? With **sex games,** stripteases and having sex in new places. Better yet if you could combine all three elements together.

Here are some ideas to help you get started:

Scenario 1: Going Away for the Weekend - If it's been a while since you went away for the weekend, this might be just what you need if things have been feeling a little lackluster lately. Take a break from your regular routine and head somewhere the two of you can be alone together. Once you arrive and settle in, it's time to head out to dinner. While your partner orders the meal, you slip away into the ladies room, take off your panties, and put them in your purse. Meanwhile, he has no idea as you make your way back to the table. The food comes, you're enjoying your meal, and then slowly slide your foot up to your partner's leg. He's surprised at first as your foot slides closer to his crotch, but then quickly reciprocates when he sees the cheeky smile you're giving him.

You slide closer as his hand travels up your leg, along the curve of your thigh until he gasps with surprise as he realized you haven't got your panties on. Whisper naughty things in his ear as his fingers begin to work their magic and when you finally feel so wet you're about to rip his clothes off, push your chair back, plant a kiss on his lips and tell him **"you know where to find me"** as you walk away seductively, swinging your hips to make sure he's got a good view of your butt as you make your way back to the room. He quickly pays for the dinners, rushes back the room, flings the door open, and is met with another happy surprise when you pull him close and push him on the bed. **"Sit there. I'm going to strip for you."**

The sexy music begins to play, you gyrate your hips slowly, turning around to make sure he can see every inch of you. You begin slowly undressing, watching his eyes grow wider and the hunger on his face becomes more apparent as you tease him with little glimpses of your flesh before letting it all drop to the floor and you're clad in nothing more than your bra and panties (which you put on again while waiting for him). Running your hands all over your body as you continue to sway to the music, move closer until you can grab him by his shirt, pull him up and whisper, **"Your turn."** By this stage, he's going to be so fired up with hormones the two of you are going to be in for a long night of lovemaking.

How to Climb Out of Your Sexual Rut

Love life feeling stale lately? That's a sign you're stuck in a sexual rut, and you'll need to work together to get out of it. Its okay to find yourself stuck; it happens even to the happiest couples. What matters is the way you work together to overcome it.

- *Talk to Each Other* - Communication is essential to overcoming this tricky stage of your relationship. But be mindful of **the way** you communicate. Avoid phrasing your words in such it way it seems like you're blaming them for the boredom you feel in the relationship. For example, don't say, **"We're stuck in a rut"** or **"The way the relationship is going right now is**

boring, don't you think?". Instead, be gentle when you communicate and say **"Let's work together and figure out what we can do."**

- *Don't Get Angry With Each Other* - The first reaction by either partner might be to feel defensive but avoid getting angry with each other. It is important to communicate honestly, and you or your partner may not feel comfortable doing that if they know it's going to make the other person mad. Then again, if you **don't** talk about it, the problem is not going to fix itself, and acknowledging that there is a problem is the first step to repairing what might need to be fixed in your relationship. Getting angry or upset about it and lashing out at each other is only going to make the situation worse. Whenever there's a problem, especially something like this involving your sex life, stay calm, talk about it and try to work things out.

- *Try Some Nonsexual Changes* - The boredom you feel might not entirely be bedroom related. Perhaps your routine together has become too mundane in general. If you suspect that might be adding to it, try making some changes or do something new together. Try a new restaurant, go for a walk together, explore a new city, go away a short getaway together. A change of routine can feel refreshing if you've been doing the same old thing day in and day out.

- *Changing Your Look* - It's not a necessity, but if it makes you feel better and gives you a confidence boost, this is one to consider. Getting a makeover can make us feel like a new and improved version of ourselves, and a shift in perspective is enough to spark a sense of excitement again. Get a haircut, get some new clothes, new makeup, whatever you feel like to boost your spirits.

- *Keep Growing and Learning* - It's hard to feel bored when you're always learning something new and growing both as an individual and a couple. Even better, take up activities you can do together, so you're **both** learning, growing, and bonding at the same time. Pick up a new hobby, read a book together, take a new class or course, learn a new skill together. There's no end to the possibilities once you start looking and discovering something new you might not have known about each other can make you see your partner in a whole new light.

Scenario 3: Little Joyful Moments- Dealing with the everyday stresses of life can suck the joy we feel if we choose to let it happen. Planning little joyful moments that are both sexual and sensual can make you feel alive again and they don't always have to be grand, romantic gestures either. Plan a candlelight dinner together. Leave love notes in their purse. Send a sexy text in the middle of the day. Deliver flowers to your partner at work. Take a relaxing bubble bath together. Have breakfast in bed this weekend. Plan a trip next month. Surprise your partner with a gift if you know they've had a hard day. There's no end to the possibilities of what you can do to. Sometimes, alleviating the boredom could be as simple as bringing a smile to your partner's face again.

Scenario 2: Hotel Role Play - Treat your next hotel stay like a naughty sex adventure, and if you want to make it even more interesting, don't tell your partner what you're up to. Make the reservations (once you've confirmed they're free of course) but don't tell your partner what you've done. Invite them to meet you at the bar for a drink. Once you spot them sitting at the bar waiting for you, get the bartender to hand them a note and the key to the room (you would have given the bartender both in advance). Surprised, your partner opens the note and sees that you've written: **"You hold the key to an erotic evening you don't want to miss. I'll be waiting".**

Your partner makes their way up to the room, heart beating a little faster in anticipation and excitement, unsure of what awaits. When they arrive, they open the door and walk into the room, looking around at their surroundings. You come up from behind, hug, and kiss them as you whisper: **"I've been fantasizing about you all day."** You then begin to recreate a sexual fantasy you know they've been eager to try out, bringing to life as you watch their eyes grow wider with surprise and delight. Tease each other, play out your dirtiest, naughtiest fantasies all night long until you're both panting heavily and basking in the warm glow of post-coital bliss.

The Stripteasing Fantasy

Spicing up your sex life is not as hard as it may seem. It's a matter of figuring out what your partner likes, what turns them on and drives them wild and going for it! A little creativity with the right visual stimulation and you're going to have a hard time holding him back as he tries to ravage you. Any red-blooded male with a healthy sex drive is bound to have several fantasies at best running through his mind. One such alluring fantasy? **Stripteasing.** The expression in your eyes, the way your body sways to the rhythm of the music, the way you taunt him by running your hands all over your body while standing just outside of reach will make him yearn for you even more. He's bound to have fantasized about you several times, but seeing his stripteasing fantasy come to life with you as the star of the show? You'll probably have to tie him down to keep him from jumping you right there and then.

You don't have to be a sexy supermodel or a porn star to turn him on and make his wild fantasy come true. The secret to turning his striptease imagery into one that is better than anything he could visualize is to tease him **throughout** the day instead of doing it right before you jump into bed together:

- Sext him throughout the day and give him a taste of what's waiting for him when he comes home tonight. Focus on toying with his imagination, revealing just enough information, so he knows what's coming.
- Practice before your big debut. Learn some dance moves that focus on a lot of hip movement and swaying that will make it hard for him to tear his eyes away from you.
- There are only three rules to stripteasing you need to remember: **Tempt, Tease and Tantalize.** Move seductively in a way that accentuates the curves of your body, focusing on your breasts and buttocks but

always tease him by staying out of reach. Close, but not close enough for him to touch. It will drive him crazy with longing for you.

- Take your stripteasing session up a notch with a pair of handcuffs or a silk scarf to tie him up. Restrict his movement and gyrate your body in front of him. If he tries to break free to grab onto you, wink seductively and tell him he's got to follow your rules. Tell him you're allowed to touch him, but **he can't touch you.** Keep gyrating your body in front of his face until he can't bear it any longer.

- Tease him by giving him a peek at the goods but no more than that. In between your dance moves and sashaying, pull your bra down so he can see a hint of a nipple. Sway your breasts in his face while you do this and then cover back up, giving him a cheeky wink as you do.

- Drop your inhibitions and lose yourself in the moment. You need to enjoy yourself as much as he enjoys watching you so your sexy dance doesn't look painfully awkward.

Other Ways to Turn Up the Heat on Your Sex Life

Sex games, role-playing and recreating fantasies can do wonders to revive the excitement you might have thought was lost in your relationship. The best part is most of the time; all you need is your imagination and some creativity. There's no end to the things you could try in the bedroom and when you're ready, let the creative, sexy time begin!

- Have sex while blindfolded and watch how your other sense comes alive. Every touch starts to feel electric and every sensation feels ten times more powerful.
- Watch porn together to bring you closer as a couple. We've all done it, **especially men,** so there's no point denying or trying to pretend like we don't. Instead of watching it solo, watch it together this time and see who gets turned on first.
- Put on a porn movie in the background and try to mimic what the couple on-screen are doing.

- Turn it into a sex game by challenging each other to see how many times a day you can have sex without repeating the same position twice.

- Go for another game where you and your lover try to do it in every room in the house and on every piece of furniture that can support you. See if you can get it done in a day, probably with an all-day sex marathon.

- Try having sex tonight using **all** the sex toys you have. Every single piece needs to be used at least once. No exceptions.

- Try dominating her in bed. 17% of women have reportedly tried bondage, and Durex's 2005 survey reported that at least 36% of adults in the United States have reportedly tried blindfolds, masks, and other bondage tools during sex. It's a huge part of the overall sexual fantasy aspect.

- Share your fantasies. Have each person write down five fantasies you would each like to role play or recreate, put them in a jar and take turns pulling one fantasy each out of the jar and get busy!

- Blindfold your partner and tease their body with different materials, textures, and sensations. Silk, feathers, whipped cream sprayed on their erogenous zones, anything you'd like as long as your partner is comfortable with it. Keep them gasping and guessing, wondering what's coming next.

- Indulge in a couple's erotic massage together if it's been a while since you've done that. Use scents that you both find relaxing and take turns helping each other relax. Make your movements nice and slow, appreciating the curves of your partner's body. Linger longer on the erogenous zones and listen to their moans as you sensually massage their sensitive areas.

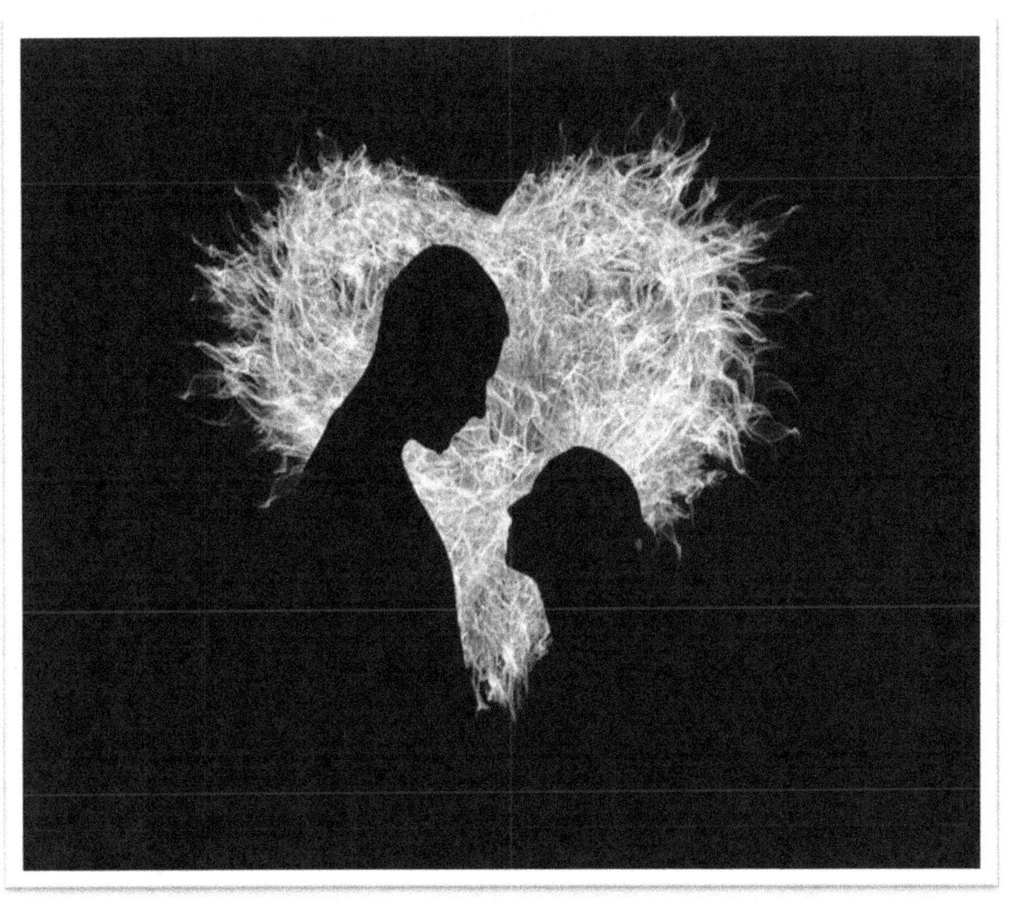

Conclusion

Just because you've finished this book doesn't mean there is nothing left to learn on the topic, expanding your horizons is the only way to find the mastery you seek. It is your sole responsibility to internalize and practice your key take always for ultimate results. You may need to break down important points and prioritize them for easy and coordinated steps to action. Once you decide to try out some of the practices discussed to ensure you understand that your partner's consent is of utmost importance as it is a critical determinant in the acquisition of pleasure and stimulation.

Start with the easy sex positions as you work your way up through intermediate ones and eventually the advanced positions. A significant first step in making sexual stimulation should be through seduction, which expresses your swish to make sexual advances. Keep in mind that it can be hard to circumvent a partner who is unwilling to try out new sex positions or explore additional sex variants. Therefore, you should approach them with respect and love and persuade them of the need for trying out something different, and it may be a step to indulge in an ecstasy of sexual stimulation and orgasm.

If you feel that you have witnessed some changes, you should keep on implementing these points and continue to repeat it. Just in case, you feel that there is not a lot of change; we want you to go through the lessons once again in the book. Make sure that you do not simply read it, implement each of them.

We have put in a questionnaire at the beginning and this is why we want you to go back to it and re-answer them. The difference should be there for you to witness. Mind-blowing sex. It is entirely possible, anywhere, anytime with the right partner and the right techniques. The basic rule of thumb to remember is to focus on stimulating your partner's senses and their bodies. This should be your primary focus, not the orgasm, and not the act of sex alone. Great sex is more than just a man and women being joined together at the genitals. It is about the chemistry, the rhythm, the compatibility, intimacy, bond and connection that they share that is unlike anything they have with anyone else. There's nothing quite like the feeling of two souls coming together as one and as the sex gets better, the relationship only grows stronger and the intimacy increases.

It comes as no surprise that when you have a happy and active sex life, you will find an overall bliss. Sex is often directly linked to happiness because ultimately we all have primal needs that we need to fulfill.

So, make the best use of this book and it is filled what too many tips and powerful lessons that are going to be of use. We have implemented these in our lives and once we were sure of the results, we presented it for your reference. So, it is upon you now to use this book the way it is meant to.

We hope that your sex drive takes a surge for the good and you get the right action in bed!